Gabriel Stux Bruce Pomeranz
Basics of Acupuncture
Third, Revised and Enlarged Edition

Springer

Berlin
Heidelberg
New York
Barcelona
Budapest
Hong Kong
London
Milan
Paris
Tokyo

Gabriel Stux   Bruce Pomeranz

Basics of
Acupuncture

Translations of Chinese Terms by K. A. Sahm
Illustrations by Petra Kofen

Third, Revised and Enlarged Edition
With 72 Figures

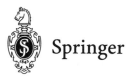 Springer

Dr. med. Gabriel Stux
Acupuncture Center
Goltsteinstraße 26, D-40211 Düsseldorf
Germany

Prof. Bruce Pomeranz MD, Ph. D
Dept. of Physiology (Faculty of Medicine)
Dept. of Zoology (Faculty of Arts and Science)
University of Toronto
25, Harbord St., Toronto M5S1A1
Ontario, Canada

This book is based on the following books published by
Springer-Verlag:

Acupuncture, Textbook and Atlas
ISBN 3-540-17331-5/0-387-17331-5

Einführung in die Akupunktur
ISBN 3-540-57453-0

ISBN 3-540-59149-4
Springer-Verlag Berlin Heidelberg NewYork

ISBN 3-540-53072-X 2nd edition Springer-Verlag Berlin Heidelberg New York
ISBN 0-387-53072-X 2nd edition Springer-Verlag New York Berlin Heidelberg

Die Deutsche Bibliothek – CIP-Einheitsaufnahme
Basics of acupuncture / Gabriel Stux ; Bruce Pomeranz. Transl. of Chinese terms
by K. A. Sahm. Ill. by Petra Kofen. – 3., rev. and enl. ed. – Berlin ; Heidelberg ;
New York : Springer, 1995
  ISBN 3-540-59149-4
NE: Stux, Gabriel; Pomeranz, Bruce

Cip Data applied for

Typesetting, printing, and binding: Appl, Wemding
SPIN: 10494617   19/3133 – 543210 – Printed on acid-free paper

Preface to the Third Edition

In 1987, our first book *Acupuncture: Textbook and Atlas* received
rave reviews (e.g., in *New England Journal of Medicine*). This
prompted us to write this smaller affordable version in order to
reach a wider audience. The smaller format has been so successful
that we are now into our third revised edition. This has given us
the opportunity to update and improve the book. For example, numerous new references to scientific advances have been added.
Also the section on traditional Chinese medicine (TCM) was added because it gives a more complete picture of the current practice of acupuncture.

Acupuncture has come a long way since our first book in 1987.
There has been a surge of interest in treating drug addictions by
ear acupuncture in 450 centers world wide. The treatment of nausea and vomiting has been so well tested (scientifically) that the
FDA (USA) is considering making this the major indication for
acupuncture in America. Research into its efficacy for neurological and pulmonary diseases is also gaining credibility. No longer is
chronic pain the only scientifically acceptable use for acupuncture
(based on the endorphin mechanism).

Finally, the exponential increase in the number of acupuncturists
worldwide (an estimated 1 million outside China) has given acupuncture the critical mass needed for its growth and survival. Indeed, many consider acupuncture to be at the forefront of alternative medicine based on acceptability by physicians, scientific valida-
tion, and its proven effectiveness. Ironically, the American legal
system in many states has overtaken the medical profession by giving convicted addicts the choice between jail and acupuncture! To
top it off the FDA (USA) is in the process of changing its 1976 rul-

ing on acupuncture from being an "experimental" to a legitimate medical procedure.

We are proud to have contributed, in some measure, to the recent success of acupuncture by writing a book which many consider to be one of the leading textbooks on the subject.

May 1995   The Authors

Preface to the First Edition

Basics of Acupuncture is an introduction to acupuncture based on several books published in German by the first author.

The chapters on the scientific basis of acupuncture and electro-acupuncture were written by Prof. Bruce Pomeranz, an eminent neurophysiologist who is in the vanguard of basic research into acupuncture, and teaches acupuncture as an elective course at University of Toronto Medical School.

Following an introduction to the philosophical and theoretical background of traditional Chinese medicine, the diagnostic system is presented. The Chinese system of channels and functional organs and the significance of the points are described. The 14 main channels with the most important acupuncture points for daily practice are presented with didactic emphasis on morphology and clinical applicability. The Chinese point names are given in the Pin Yin Transcription according to the latest standardization of the World Health Organization and are translated by Karl Alfried Sahm into English.

The methods of needling and moxibustion are described in detail with their clinical applications. The chapter on treatment is based on Western modes of diagnosis, discussed in relation to Chinese diagnostic categories, and the major principles of therapy. The most important acupuncture points are given for the different diagnoses. They should *not be used as "recipes"* but as hints to which underlying rules should be used for the selection of points.

For a more detailed book the reader ist referred to the standard textbook: *Acupuncture Textbook and Atlas* by the same authors (Springer-Verlag ISBN 3-540-17331-5).

Thanks are due to Prof. A. Jayasuriya, Dr. Maria Vinnemeier, Prof. Zhang Jin, and Prof. Cheng Xingnong who have had important influences on this book. Thanks to Britta Severin, Janet Dodsworth and Alison Fisher for translation work and for correction of the manuscript.

Spring, 1988   Gabriel Stux

Table of Contents

1	**Introduction** (B. Pomeranz)	1
	Growth of Clinical Acupuncture in the West	2
2	**Scientific Basis of Acupuncture** (B. Pomeranz)	4
2.1	Acupuncture Analgesia (Basic Research)	4
2.1.1	Neural Mechanisms of Acupuncture Analgesia	5
2.1.2	Evidence for Endorphins and Acupuncture Analgesia	13
2.1.3	Evidence for Midbrain Monoamines and Acupuncture Analgesia	18
2.1.4	Evidence for Pituitary Hypothalamic System and Acupuncture Analgesia	19
2.1.5	Conclusions	20
2.2	Acupuncture Analgesia for Chronic Pain	21
2.3	Drug Addiction	24
2.4	Nerve Regeneration, Cardiovascular, Antiemetic and Urogenital Effects of Acupuncture	26
2.5	Acupuncture Points (Do They Really Exist?)	28
2.5.1	Does Needling at True Points Work Better Than Needling at Sham Points?	29
2.5.2	Are There Unique Anatomical Structures at Acupuncture Points?	30
2.5.3	Do Acupuncture Points Have Unique Physiological Features?	32
2.5.4	What Nerves Are Activated by Acupuncture?	36
3	**Background and Theory of Traditional Chinese Medicine** (G. Stux)	61
3.1	Tao, Yin, and Yang	61
3.2	The Vital Energy, Life Force: Qi	62

3.3	Pathogenesis of Chinese Medicine	64
3.4	The System of Five Phases	66
3.5	Diagnosis in Traditional Chinese Medicine	67
4	**Channels, Organs, and Points** (G. Stux)	72
4.1	System of Channels and Organs	72
4.2	Point Categories	78
4.2.1	Shu Points or Transport Points	78
4.2.2	Mu or Alarm Points	78
4.2.3	Influential Points, Hui Xue	79
4.2.4	Xi-Cleft Points	79
4.2.5	Five Shu Points	79
4.2.6	Tonification Point	80
4.2.7	Sedative Point	80
4.2.8	Jing Well Point	80
4.2.9	Ying Point	80
4.2.10	Yuan Source Point	81
4.2.11	Jing Point	81
4.2.12	He Sea Point	81
4.2.13	Luo Connecting Point	82
4.2.14	Confluent Points	82
4.3	Methods of Point Location	82
4.4	Description of Channels and Points	88
4.4.1	Lung Channel	88
4.4.2	Large Intestine Channel	96
4.4.3	Stomach Channel	102
4.4.4	Spleen Channel	112
4.4.5	Heart Channel	118
4.4.6	Small Intestine Channel	122
4.4.7	Urinary Bladder Channel	126
4.4.8	Kidney Channel	140
4.4.9	Pericardium Channel	144
4.4.10	Sanjiao Channel	148
4.4.11	Gallbladder Channel	154
4.4.12	Liver Channel	164
4.4.13	Du Mai	168
4.4.14	Ren Mai	174
4.4.15	Extra Points	180

5	**Technique of Acupuncture** (G. Stux)	188
5.1	Acupuncture Needles	188
5.2	De Qi Sensation	190
5.3	Tonifying and Sedating Methods of Stimulation	191
5.4	Sterilization of the Needles	192
5.5	Complications of Acupuncture Treatment	193
5.6	Moxibustion	194
5.7	Acupressure	197
5.8	Laser Acupuncture	198
6	**Acupuncture Treatment** (G. Stux)	200
6.1	Principles of Acupuncture and Rules of Point Selection	201
6.2	**Locomotor Disorders**	209
6.2.1	Cervical Spondylitis, Torticollis, Rheumatoid Arthritis	209
6.2.2	Intercostal Neuralgia, Trauma of the Thorax,	
	Ankylosing Spondylitis, Zoster Neuralgia	210
6.2.3	Sciatica, Lumbar Pain	211
6.2.4	Periarthritis Humeroscapularis, Frozen Shoulder	212
6.2.5	Epicondylitis, Tennis Elbow	213
6.2.6	Coxarthrosis, Coxarthritis	214
6.2.7	Gonarthrosis, Pain in the Knee Joint	214
6.2.8	Rheumatoid Arthritis	215
6.3	**Respiratory Disorders**	217
6.3.1	Common Cold	218
6.3.2	Maxillary Sinusitis	219
6.3.3	Frontal Sinusitis	219
6.3.4	Chronic Bronchitis	220
6.3.5	Bronchial Asthma	220
6.4	**Cardiovascular Disorders**	222
6.4.1	Coronary Heart Disease with Angina Pectoris	222
6.4.2	Cardiac Neurosis	222
6.4.3	Exhaustion Conditions in Heart Disease	223
6.4.4	Hypertension	223
6.4.5	Hypotension	224
6.4.6	Disturbances of Peripheral Blood Supply	224

6.5   Gastroenterological Disorders   225
6.5.1   Gastritis, Gastroenteritis   226
6.5.2   Gastric and Duodenal Ulcers   226
6.5.3   Diarrhea   227
6.5.4   Irritable Bowel Disease   228
6.5.5   Constipation   229
6.5.6   Cholangitis, Cholecystitis, Biliary Dyskinesia,
        Biliary Colic   229

6.6   Mental Disturbances and Illnesses   230
6.6.1   Depression   230
6.6.2   Exhaustion Conditions   232
6.6.3   Agitation   232
6.6.4   Sleep Disturbances   233
6.6.5   Drug Addiction   233
6.6.6   Alcohol Addiction   235
6.6.7   Nicotine Addiction   235
6.6.8   Overweight, Weight Loss   236

6.7   Neurological Disorders   237
6.7.1   Headache and Migraine   237
6.7.2   Trigeminal Neuralgia   239
6.7.3   Hemiparesis   240
6.7.4   Facial Paresis   242
6.7.5   Epilepsy   242

6.8   Gynecological Disorders   244
6.8.1   Dysmenorrhea   244
6.8.2   Pain Caused by Gynecological Tumors   245
6.8.3   Analgesia During Childbirth   245

6.9   Urological Disorders   247
6.9.1   Pyelonephritis, Urinary Infections, Chronic
        Glomerulonephritis   248
6.9.2   Prostatitis, Psychogenic Urological Symptoms   248
6.9.3   Enuresis   249

6.10   Skin Disorders   250
6.10.1 Acne Vulgaris   250
6.10.2 Leg Ulcers, Deficient Wound Healing   251

6.10.3 Eczema, Neurodermatitis 252
6.10.4 Psoriasis 252
6.10.5 Herpes Simplex 252

6.11 **Disorders of the Sense Organs** 253
6.11.1 Deafness 253
6.11.2 Tinnitus 253
6.11.3 Ménière's Syndrome, Dizziness, Motion Sickness,
       Labyrinthitis 254
6.11.4 Chronic Conjunctivitis 254
6.11.5 Visual Deficiency 255

6.12 **Acute Disorders and Emergencies** 256
6.12.1 Fainting, Collapse 256
6.12.2 Epileptic Fits, Grand Mal 257
6.12.3 Acutely Painful Conditions 257

7   **Electroacupuncture and Transcutaneous Electrical
        Nerve Stimulation** (B. Pomeranz) 258
7.1   Electroacupuncture 258
7.2   Transcutaneous Electrical Nerve Stimulation,
       TENS 263
7.3   Acupuncture-like TENS Differs from Conventional
       TENS 265
7.4   Habituation to Monotonous Stimuli 268

8   **Traditional Chinese Syndromes:
        The Diagnosis of Chinese Medicine** (G. Stux) 269
8.1   Major Patterns of Disturbances 270
8.2   Syndromes of the Five Zang Organs 272
8.3   The Most Frequent Syndromes 275

9   **Additional Methods of Treatment** (G. Stux) 283
9.1   Chakra Acupuncture 283
9.2   Awareness Release Technique 290

Appendixes A–D (G. Stux)

A. World Health Organization
   List of Indications for Acupuncture 293
B. Nomenclature and Abbreviations for Channels and Points 294

C. Glossary of Chinese Terms 296
D. Alphabetic List of Chinese Point Names 300

Bibliography 305

Introduction

B. POMERANZ

Acupuncture was first brought into Europe in the 17th century, but until recently was not widely accepted because of a clash of paradigms, East versus West. Chinese medicine is based on holistic patterns, acausal relationships, nonlinear logic, and non-reductionistic phenomenology. Western medicine (in contrast) is based on linear causality and reductionistic scientific theories. Western medical science is quick to reject a phenomenon if it does not fit the current scientific theories. Chinese Taoism had a distaste for explanatory theories and chose instead merely to observe phenomena in order to be in harmony with mother nature. If a needle in the hand cured a toothache, that was sufficient for Chinese Taoism. For Western medicine acupuncture was impossible and hence was relegated to the wastebasket of placebo effects.

For years Western sceptics argued that the evidence for acupuncture was merely anecdotal. However, as described in Chap. 2, this situation has drastically changed in the past 10 years. Controlled clinical trials on chronic pain have proved that acupuncture helps from 55% to 85% of patients, while placebo controls benefit only 30%–35% of cases. Moreover, hundreds of rigorous publications (in many leading Western journals) have revealed the reductionistic, causal mechanisms for many of the acupuncture effects (e.g., release of endorphins, serotonin, cortisol).

Growth of Clinical Acupuncture in the West

Scientific advances in acupuncture research coupled with the side effects of treating chronic pain by conventional drugs have promoted acupuncture usage dramatically in the last decade. It is estimated that over one million practitioners outside China administer acupuncture treatment for chronic pain, and of these, over 300000 are physicians. In a recent study of German pain clinics, it was found that 90% of the physicians used acupuncture. In the USA there are over 11000 physicians (MDs and DOs) with an interest in acupuncture (J. Helms, personal communication). Over 2000 Canadian physicians have taken courses given by the Acupuncture Foundation of Canada (L. Rapson, personal communication). Moreover, veterinarians, chiropractors, and naturopaths use acupuncture even more than physicians in North America. In addition there are numerous practitioners exclusively using acupuncture (there are 16 schools in the United States that are accredited by the Federal Government giving 4-year courses in acupuncture to non-physicians).

Because acupuncture is new in America, the regulations governing its use are in a state of flux. There are five categories of regulations:

1. Eleven states require a certain number of hours of acupuncture training (or the passing of an examination) by licenced physicians before they can practise acupuncture: California, District of Columbia, Georgia, Illinois, Louisiana, Maryland, Montana, New York, Nevada, Pennsylvania, and Virginia.
2. In 18 states acupuncture is considered the practice of medicine without further training and is restricted to licenced physicians: Alabama, Alaska, Arkansas, Idaho, Indiana, Iowa, Kansas, Kentucky, Michigan, Mississippi, Missouri, New Hampshire, North Carolina, North Dakota, Ohio, South Dakota, West Virginia, and Wyoming.
3. Twelve states independently license or register non-physician acupuncturists based on training and/or examinations: California, District of Columbia, Florida, Hawaii, Montana, Nevada,

New Mexico, New Jersey, New York, Oregon, Rhode Island, and Washington.

4. Four states license or register acupuncturists under some sort of medical (MD) supervision (e.g., referral from an MD): Maryland, Massachusetts, Pennsylvania, and Utah.

5. Ten states only allow acupuncturists to practise under close medical (MD) supervision: Arizona, Colorado, Connecticut, Delaware, Louisiana, Maine, Tennessee, Texas, Vermont, and Wisconsin.

(N.B. Three states do not fit any of these five categories.)

Despite this growing recognition of acupuncture by physicians and by state legislatures, the US Federal Food and Drug Administration (FDA) considers acupuncture to be an experimental procedure, and hence all acupuncture devices are placed in category 3 (for experimental devices). This currently being revised. This contrasts with the recent ruling of a Texas judge who stated that if acupuncture was an experimental way of doing medicine, then the Chinese language was an experimental way of talking!

Similar confusion exists among health insurance schemes in America, some of which cover acupuncture and others which do not. It often depends on individual corporations or trade unions and their demand for coverage. In Ontario (Canada), the government medical insurance scheme covers acupuncture, but at a relatively low fee.

Despite the confusion, this is an exciting time for acupuncturists. While many cities have an oversupply of physicians with insufficient work, most good acupuncturists have long waiting lists. Perhaps the patients will be the final arbitrators!

2 Scientific Basis of Acupuncture

B. POMERANZ

In this chapter some of the modern scientific studies on acupuncture are outlined. A more detailed review appears in *Acupuncture Textbook and Atlas* by Stux and Pomeranz [179a] and *Scientific Bases of Acupuncture* by Pomeranz and Stux [151a].

2.1 Acupuncture Analgesia (Basic Research)

In recent years in the west, acupuncture analgesia (AA) has been restricted mainly to the treatment of chronic pain and has not been used for surgical procedures except for demonstration purposes. In some Western countries, however, AA is used in combination with nitrous oxide (sufficient N_2O being given to render the patient unconscious, but not enough for analgesia) [76] or with fentanyl [83b]. However, even for the treatment of chronic pain, many Western physicians were sceptical at first, despite a vast body of anecdotal evidence from both China and Europe.

How could a needle in the hand possibly relieve a toothache? Because such phenomena did not conform to physiological concepts, scientists were puzzled and sceptical. Many explained it by the well-known placebo effect which works through suggestion, distraction, or even hypnosis [199, 200]. In 1945 Beecher [11] had shown that morphine relieved pain in 70% of patients, while sugar injections (placebo) reduced pain in 35% of patients who *believed* they were receiving morphine. Thus, many medical scientists in the early 1970s assumed that AA worked by the placebo (psychological) effect. However, there were several problems with this idea. How does one explain the use of AA in veterinary medicine over the past 1000 years in China and for approximately 100 years in Europe, and its growing use on animals in America? Animals are not suggestible, and only a very few species are capable of the still reaction (so-called animal hypnosis). Similarly, small children respond to AA. Moreover, several studies in which patients were given psychological tests for suggestibility did not show a good correlation between AA and suggestibility [98]. Hypnosis has also been ruled out as an explanation, as there have been two studies [7, 61] showing that hypnosis and AA respond differently to naloxone, AA being blocked and hypnosis being unaffected by this endorphin antagonist.

Up to 1973 the evidence for AA was mainly anecdotal, with a huge collection of case histories from one-quarter of the world's population. Unfortunately, there were few scientifically controlled experiments to convince the sceptics. In the past 17 years, however, the situation has changed considerably. Scientists have been asking two important questions. First, does AA really work (that is by a physiological rather than a placebo/psychological effect)? Second, if it does work, what is the mechanism?

The first question (does it work?) had to be approached by way of controlled experiments to remove placebo effects, spontaneous remissions, etc. These have been carried out in clinical practice on patients with chronic pain (see Sect. 2.2), in the laboratory on humans, studying acute laboratory-induced pain (see Sect. 2.5), and on animals (see Sect. 2.5). From these numerous studies it can be concluded that AA works much better than placebo.

Hence AA must have some physiological basis. But what are the possible mechanisms? Only the answer to the second question (how does AA work?) could possibly dispel the deep scepticism toward acupuncture.

2.1.1 Neural Mechanisms of Acupuncture Analgesia

Ten years of research in my laboratory, coupled with over a hundred papers from the western scientific literature led to a compelling hypothesis: AA is initiated by stimulation of small diameter nerves in muscles, which send impulses to the spinal cord, and then three centers, spinal cord, midbrain, and pituitary, are activated to release transmitter chemicals (endorphins and monoamines) which block "pain" messages. Figures 1 and 2 summarize various aspects of the hypothesis of the neural mechanism of AA. First we explain the figures, and then present some of the evidence for the hypothesis. Figure 1 shows how pain messages are transmitted from the skin to the cerebral cortex. On the left is skin with a muscle beneath it in the lower left corner. An acupuncture needle penetrates the muscle. The next rectangle is spinal cord, and to the right are rectangles depicting various brain structures: midbrain, thalamus, pituitary-hypothalamus, and cerebral cortex. As shown in the legend to Fig. 1, open triangles represent excitatory terminals (acting at the synapse) and closed triangles, inhibitory terminals. Large arrows indicate the direction of flow of impulses in the axons and small arrow, the painful stimulus.

In order to understand the pain transmission shown in Fig. 1, follow the thick arrows at the top. An injury to the skin activates the sensory receptors of small afferent nerve fibers (labelled 1) of A delta and C axon size. (Nerve fibers are classified by size and according to whether they originate in skin or muscle: large diameter myelinated nerves A beta [skin] or type I [muscle] carry "touch" and proprioception, respectively. Small diameter myelinated A delta [skin] or types II and III [muscle] carry "pain"; the smallest unmyelinated C [skin] and type IV [muscle] also carry "pain". Types II, III, IV and C also carry nonpainful messages.) Cell 1 synapses onto the STT (spinothalamic tract) cell in the spinal cord (labelled 2). The STT (cell 2) projects its axon to the thalamus to synapse onto cell 3, which sends impulses to the cortex to activate cell 4 (probably in the primary somatosensory cortex). I must point out that this diagram is oversimplified, since there are at least six possible pathways carrying painful messages from the spinal cord to the cortex, but for the sake of clarity only the STT is shown.

For the other cells (cells 5–14) it is best to go to Fig. 2 to see how they operate. In Fig. 2, the acupuncture needle is shown activating a sensory receptor (square) inside the muscle, and this sends impulses to the spinal cord via the cell labelled 5, which represents

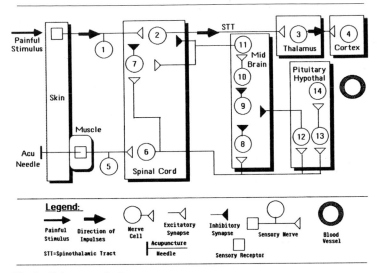

Fig. 1. Pain transmission

type II and III muscle afferent nerves (small diameter myelinated afferents). Type II afferents are thought to signal the numbness of De Qi needling sensations and type III, the fullness (heaviness and mild aching) sensation [201]. If soreness is also felt, that is carried by unmyelinated type IV afferents from the muscle (but soreness is not usually part of the De Qi sensations). In some acupuncture points there are no muscles (e. g., at the finger tips, over major nerve trunks), and here different fibers are involved. (If cutaneous nerves are activated, the A delta fibers are the relevant ones.) Cell number 5 synapses in the spinal cord onto an ALT (anterolateral tract) cell (labelled 6) which projects to three centers; the spinal cord, the midbrain, and the pituitary-hypothalamic complex.

Within the spinal cord, cell 6 sends a short segmental branch to cell 7, which is an endorphinergic cell. This cell releases either enkephalin or dynorphin, but not β-endorphin. (There are three families of endorphins: enkephalin, β-endorphin and dynorphin, and these are all labelled E in Fig. 2.) The spinal cord endorphins cause presynaptic inhibition of cell 1 (preventing transmission of the painful message from cell 1 to cell 2). As there are very few axo-

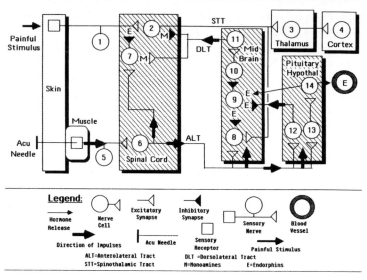

Fig. 2. Acupuncture (low frequency, high intensity)

axonal synapses between cell 7 and cell 1, it is thought that the endorphin peptides merely diffuse to the receptors located on the terminals of cell 1. There are also postsynaptic endorphin synapses acting directly onto cell 2 from cell 7, though these are not shown. Thus, enkephalins and dynorphins block pain transmission at the spinal cord level. The presynaptic inhibition probably works by reducing calcium current inflow during the action potential in the terminals of cell 1, resulting in reduced release of the pain transmitter.

What Fig. 2 does not show are the numerous peptides present in the terminals of cell 1 (among these are cholecystokinin, somatostatin, neurotensin, bombesin, calcitonin gene-related peptide, angiotensin, substance P, and vasoactive intestinal peptide). So far only cholecystokinin (CCK) has been shown to play a role in AA [71], acting like naloxone, the opiate antagonist, to block endorphin-mediated AA (perhaps the ratio of CCK and endorphins is the important variable in producing analgesia). The roles of the other peptides in pain and analgesia are not known, partly because good antagonists are not available to study them.

As shown in Fig. 2 cell 6 also projects to the midbrain, ascending the spinal cord in the ALT. Here it excites cells in the periaqueductal grey (PAG; cells 8 and 9), which release enkephalin to disinhibit cell 10 (which is thus excited) and in turn activates the raphe nucleus (the raphe nucleus is located in the caudal end of the medulla oblongata [cell 11]), causing it to send impulses down the dorsolateral tract (DLT) to release monoamines (serotonin and norepinephrine; labelled M) onto the spinal cord cells [67]. Cell 2 is inhibited by postsynaptic inhibition, while cell 1 is presynaptically inhibited via cell 7 (cell 7 is excited while cell 2 is inhibited by the monoamines). Either of the two monoamine mechanisms can suppress the pain transmission. In addition to the raphe magnus, which releases serotonin onto the cord, there is the adjacent reticularis paragigantocellularis (not shown), which may release norepinephrine via the DLT onto the spinal cord (norepinephrine binds to an alpha receptor in the cord to block pain transmission). Some believe that serotonin and norepinephrine act synergistically in this regard [65]. There is some evidence that the peptide neurotensin may be the excitatory transmitter between cells 10 and 11 [9]. The precise relationship of these descending monoamine effects to AA is not clear at present, and results suggest that some of the raphe serotonin effect in AA may be mediated by ascending fibers from the raphe to the forebrain (not shown). More work is needed on the role of the monoamine system in AA.

Even less well understood is the action of cell 6 onto cells 12 and 13 (the pituitary hypothalamic complex). Cell 12 in the arcuate nucleus may activate the raphe via β-endorphin, and cell 13 in the hypothalamus may release β-endorphin from the pituitary gland from cell 14 (see Fig. 2). While there is some agreement that AA is accompanied by elevated β-endorphin in the CSF [175] (and blood) and that pituitary lesions suppress AA [34], there is no agreement on how the β-endorphin from the pituitary reaches the brain to cause analgesia. Too little reaches the blood to cross the blood-brain barrier in sufficient quantities. Some evidence suggests that the pituitary-portal venous system can carry hormones in a retrograde direction directly to the brain [13]. Perhaps cell 14 can influence cell 9 as shown by the thin arrows (Fig. 2), without having to cross the blood-brain barrier. If so, the role of circulating endorphins in the blood is unclear. However there is an important correlate of pituitary β-endorphin release: adrenocorticotrophic hormone (ACTH) and β-endorphin are both coreleased on an equimolar basis into the circulation [161] (they are both made from a common precursor). The ACTH travels to the adrenal cortex, where cortisol is released into the blood [35], which may explain why acupuncture is helpful in blocking the inflammation of arthritis and the bronchospasms of asthma (the doses of cortisol released by acupuncture are small and finely regulated, thus avoiding the side effects of cortisol drug therapy). (Because of insufficient data other centers implicated in the AA-endorphin effects have been left out: these include the nucleus accumbens, amygdala, habenula, and anterior caudate [74b, 224].) In Fig.2 the axon from the STT cell (cell 2) has a collateral fiber dropping down to excite cell 8 in the midbrain to cause analgesia. This is because in 1979, Le Bars et al. [90b] discovered a phenomenon called DNIC (diffuse noxious inhibitory control), in which one pain inhibits another. Its role in AA has been suggested but never clearly established [13a].

In summary, acupuncture stimulates nerve fibers in the muscle, which send impulses to the spinal cord and activates three centers (spinal cord, midbrain, and hypothalamus-pituitary) to cause analgesia. The *spinal* site uses enkephalin and dynorphin to block incoming messages with stimulation at low frequency and other transmitters (perhaps gamma-aminobutyric acid, GABA), with stimulation at high frequency. The *midbrain* uses enkephalin to activate the raphe descending system, which inhibits spinal cord pain transmission by a synergistic effect of the monoamines, serotonin, and norepinephrine. The midbrain also has a circuit which bypasses the endorphinergic links at high-frequency stimulation. Finally, at the third center, the *hypothalamus-pituitary,* the pituitary releases β-endorphin into the blood and CSF to cause analgesia at a distance. Also, the hypothalamus sends long axons to the midbrain and via β-endorphin activates the descending analgesia system. This third center is activated not at high-frequency, but only at low-frequency stimulation.

What is the practical significance of this three-level system? When needles are placed close to the site of pain or in the tender (trigger, or Ah Shi) points, they are maximizing the segmental circuits operating at cell 7 within the spinal cord, while also bringing in cells 11 and 14 in the other two centers (Fig. 2). When needles are placed in distal points far away from the painful region, they activate the midbrain and hypothalamus-pituitary (cells 11 and 14) without the benefit of local segmental effects at cell 7. Moreover, cells 11 and 14 produce analgesia throughout the body, while cell 7 produces analgesia only locally.

Local segmental needling usually gives a more intensive analgesia than distal nonsegmental needling, because it uses all three centers. Generally, the two kinds of needling (local and distal) are used together on each patient, to enhance one another. Another important practical consequence of this system is the frequency/intensity effect. As shown in Fig. 2, low-frequency (2–4 Hz), high-intensity needling works through the endorphin system and acts in all three centers, while a high-frequency (50–200 Hz), low-intensity needling only activates cells 7 and 11, bypassing the endorphin system. Numerous studies have shown that the types of analgesia produced by these two approaches are quite different [3]: the low-frequency method produces an analgesia of slower onset, and more importantly, of long duration, outlasting the 20-min stimulation session by 30 min to many hours. Also, its effects are cumulative, becoming increasingly better after several treatments. The high-frequency, low-intensity analgesia, in contrast, is rapid in onset but of very short duration, with no cumulative effects. Many authors have arbitrarily described the low-frequency, high-intensity type of analgesia as "acupuncture-like" TENS, when it is produced with transcutaneous electrical nerve stimulation, and the high-frequency, low-intensity type as "conventional" TENS.

Because low-frequency, high-intensity analgesia produces a cumulative effect, repeated treatments produce more and more benefit for the patient [111, 156, 198] or laboratory animal [152]. This could be due to long-lasting effects of endorphins in the low-frequency system. Most conventional TENS (high-frequency) devices must be worn continuously by the patients, as the effect is of short duration, and in over 70% of cases the effectiveness wears off after some months of continuous use because tolerance develops [211]. In contrast, low-frequency acupuncture need only be given daily (or twice a week), because of its long-term cumulative effects [156]. Indeed, too frequent application of low-frequency acupuncture produces tolerance; for example, if applied continuously for 6 h, the analgesia weakens and then disappears [70]. This effect is cross-tolerant with morphine tolerance [70], and the mechanisms involved may be similar to those of addiction to endorphins. Hence, spacing the acupuncture treatments with long enough intervals may prevent tolerance while promoting the cumulative effects. Perhaps the failure of some Western clinics to achieve success is due to the use of very infrequent treatment (e.g., 1 per week) and the termination of treatment after only five to ten sessions. In some clinics in Asia patients are treated daily for a month, then weekly for 6 months, and the results reported anecdotally are excellent. Of course, some patients will never respond to acupuncture for various reasons: nonresponders may be genetically deficient in opiate receptors; we have shown that mice genetically lacking endorphin receptors respond poorly to acupuncture [138]. Other failures may be due to deficiency in endorphin molecules: rats lacking endorphin compounds respond poorly to acupuncture [126]. Some non-responders can be converted to responders by treatment with the safe drug D-phenylalanine which potentiates endorphins [31, 49]. In clinical practice a strategy must be developed to allow nonresponders to be recognized while not aborting therapy too soon for potential responders who might show delayed cumulative effects. (One way is to decide after five treatments: if there is no benefit whatsoever, abort; if mild to moderate effects occur continue and reassess after 10–15 treatments.) Often the cost of repeated office visits is prohibitive. Hence, our group had developed a home acupuncture-like TENS device (which gives De Qi sensations): this can be used over acupuncture points by the patient for 30 min a day for several months [33] (see Chap. 7).

Most textbooks might have ended this discussion of AA right here. However, because acupuncture is so controversial and relatively new to Western medicine, more data are needed to convince the student that the acupuncture mechanisms outlined in Figs. 1 and 2 are well established. Those who are in a hurry can skim or skip the next few pages but should nonetheless scrutinize the reference list (this omits the huge literature from China which, if included, would double the number of citations). It should be apparent that we know more about AA than about many chemical drugs in routine use (for example, we know very little about the mechanisms of action of most anesthetic gases, but we use them regularly). The reader is also referred to recent reviews [67, 68b, 74a, 81c, 94a, 120, 143, 146, 151a, 179a, 216a, 223d, 225a].

2.1.2 Evidence for Endorphins and Acupuncture Analgesia

Perhaps the most exciting experiments, which opened up the field of AA to scientific research, were those in which endorphin antagonists (e.g., naloxone, naltrexone) were used. That naloxone could antagonize AA was reported initially by two groups [116, 149]. Mayer et al. [116], studying acute laboratory-induced tooth pain in human volunteers, produced AA by manual twirling of needles in LI.4 (first dorsal interosseus muscle of the hand). In a double-blind design they gave one group of subjects i.v. naloxone, while another group received i.v. saline. The saline group achieved AA with a time-course typical of clinical reports (30 min to onset of analgesia and effects lasting for over 1 h). The naloxone-treated group showed no AA. As there were no controls receiving naloxone alone, one might argue that naloxone hyperalgesia simply subtracted from the analgesia of AA. However, this is probably not the case, since numerous studies on acute laboratory-induced pain have shown that naloxone alone rarely produces hyperalgesia [60]. (This suggests that endorphins do not have a basal tone during acute pain.) Mayer et al. [116] also studied a control group of subjects receiving placebo injections. The placebo subjects were told to expect a strong analgesic effect, and none was observed (as predicted from Beecher's work on acute pain, where only 3% of subjects reported placebo analgesia [11]).

The other early naloxone study was by Pomeranz and Chiu [149] in awake mice; they used the mouse squeak latency paradigm and gave EA at LI.4. Numerous control groups were used in this latter experiment in an attempt to pick out some of the possible artifacts. Each group received one of the following treatments: EA alone, EA plus saline, EA plus i.v. naloxone, sham EA in a non-acupuncture point, naloxone alone, saline alone, or no treatment at all (just handling, restraint, and repeated pain testing). The results were unequivocal: naloxone completely blocked AA; sham EA produced no effect; and naloxone alone produced very little hyperalgesia (not enough to explain reduction of AA by subtraction). Moreover, the results in mice and in humans indicated, first, that AA was not a psychological effect and secondly, that AA was truly blocked by naloxone. In a later study, Cheng and Pomeranz [29] produced a dose-response curve for naloxone and found that increasing doses produced increasing blockade. In a third study in anesthetized cats, Pomeranz and Cheng [148], recording from layer-5 cells in the spinal cord (cell 2 in Fig. 1), completely prevented the EA effects with i. v. naloxone.

Since these early papers there have been numerous studies in which systemically administered endorphin antagonists have been used to test the endorphin-AA hypothesis. Although most researchers reported naloxone antagonism [17, 21, 25, 29–31, 39, 53, 63, 75, 88, 91 b, 92, 136, 138, 148, 149, 152, 166, 172, 173, 176, 177, 181, 189, 194, 210, 213, 224, 225], a few did not find any effects of naloxone [1, 23, 24, 140, 187, 198, 214]. Three of these seven failures were obtained with high-frequency, low-intensity stimulation, which is probably not endorphinergic [1, 198, 214]. In one of the failures [24] low-intensity stimulation was used, which did not lead to De Qi sensations: in spite of this four of seven subjects in that study showed naloxone antagonism. While the reasons for the other three negative papers [23, 140, 187] are not entirely clear, a possible explanation has recently emerged. Antagonists work best when given before the treatment [147, 202] and fail to reverse analgesia that has already been initiated. Thus, naloxone can prevent but often cannot reverse AA. (In the three failed experiments researchers tried to reverse AA, giving the endorphin antagonist after, not before, the acupuncture treatments.) Taken together, the overwhelming weight of evidence shows that naloxone antagonizes AA and that the few negative results may be due to poor timing of the naloxone administration. In biology, negative results are often less valid than positive results.

A few weeks after the first naloxone results were announced in the research news section of *Science* [112], a letter to the editor in the same journal justifiably criticized the use of naloxone as the

14

sole proof of the AA-endorphin hypothesis [74]. This criticism is based mainly on the argument that naloxone is a drug that might possess unknown side effects (unrelated to opiate receptor blocking). Small doses which were effective in preventing AA (in man 5×10^{-8} M, in mice and cats 10^{-6} M) would tend to implicate receptor effects: but the effectiveness of small doses of naloxone is clearly not enough evidence to prove specificity [168]. However, since that letter was written 15 different lines of experimentation have emerged which have independently provided support for the AA-endorphin hypothesis:

1. Four different opiate antagonists block AA [26a, 29].
2. Naloxone has a stereospecific effect [29].
3. Microinjection of naloxone (or antibodies to endorphins) blocks AA only if given into analgesic sites in the central nervous system [13b, 38, 68, 71, 72, 136, 147, 152, 217, 223b, 224].
4. Mice genetically deficient in opiate receptors show poor AA [138, 162].
5. Rats deficient in endorphin show poor AA [126, 181].
6. Endorphin levels rise in blood and CSF during AA and fall in specific brain regions during AA [6a, 38, 50, 73a, 74b, 78b, 85, 109, 113, 129, 139, 175, 196, 225].
7. AA is enhanced by protecting endorphins from enzyme degradation [31, 38, 49, 54, 64, 78, 126, 181, 225].
8. AA can be transmitted to a second animal by CSF transfer or by cross-circulation, and this effect is blocked by naloxone [92, 105, 159].
9. Reduction of pituitary endorphins suppresses AA [34, 113, 153, 182a, 182c–e].
10. There was a rise in messenger RNA for proenkephalin in brain and pituitary: this lasted 24–48 h after 30 min of EA indicating a prolonged increased rate of synthesis of enkephalin. This could explain the enduring effects of EA and the potentiation of repeated daily treatments [223a].
11. There is cross-tolerance between AA and morphine analgesia, implicating endorphins in AA [26a, 70].
12. AA is more effective against emotional aspects of pain; this is typical of endorphins [218a].

13. Lesions of the arcuate nucleus of hypothalamus (the site of β-endorphins) abolishes AA; this is cell 12 in Fig. 2 [182a, 182b, 201a].
14. Lesions of the periaquaductal gray (site of endorphins) abolishes AA [201b].
15. The level of c-*fos* gene protein (which measures increased neural activity) is elevated in endorphin-related areas of the brain during AA [91a].

In summary, 16 different lines of research (the 15 listed plus the naloxone studies) strongly support the AA-endorphin hypothesis. With so much convergent evidence for this hypothesis, why are there still a few sceptics?

1. Some sceptics cite the few failures of naloxone to reverse AA [24]. It has already been suggested (above) that naloxone reversal experiments are prone to difficulty because naloxone prevents but does not reverse AA. Moreover, the number of successful naloxone antagonisms of AA far exceeds the number of failures (28 successes versus 7 failures). In general, negative results are less reliable than positive results in biomedical research.
2. Sceptics state that naloxone antagonism is necessary but not sufficient evidence [74]. That is why we have presented ten *different* lines of evidence (only one line of evidence depends on naloxone).
3. Some sceptics attack animal studies of AA as being unrelated to AA in humans [24]. First, there have been numerous experiments in humans which have had the same AA-endorphin outcome as in lower animals, Second, the similarity of results across many species proves the generality of the phenomenon. Third, there is no proper objective measure of pain in man. Fourth, if sceptics are correct, then the entire animal "pain" literature should be discarded, a literature which gave us our initial insights into endorphins, brain stimulation analgesia, TENS, and other results that have been highly applicable to human pain.
4. Some sceptics are concerned that AA in animals may merely be stress-induced analgesia (which also releases endorphins) and hence has nothing to do with acupuncture in humans [24]. At a recent conference on stress-induced analgesia at the New York

Academy of Sciences we gave a lecture entitled: "Relation of stress-induced analgesia to acupuncture analgesia." Some of the points made in that paper [144] were:

- Sham EA on nearby nonacupuncture points in animals induces no AA, thus controlling for stress [19, 35, 55, 56, 99, 149, 182, 188].
- AA elicited in anesthetized rats and cats, or decerebrate cats, does not involve psychological stress [19, 55, 56, 137, 147, 148, 150, 152, 153, 188].
- AA at one frequency is endorphin mediated, while at another it is serotonin mediated, yet both give similar levels of stress [30, 176].
- Many mechanisms of stress analgesia are very different from those of AA.
- Results in mice and rats were obtained with mild stimulation activating A beta nerve fibers, a nonpainful procedure which is no more stressful than sham point stimulation [136, 151, 188].

In conclusion, the objections raised by a few sceptics are easily refuted. The overwhelming evidence supports the AA-endorphin hypothesis.

Zhang [223d] recently reviewed other differences between AA and stress analgesia:

- AA is naloxone reversible, but stress analgesia is only partly antagonized by large doses of naloxone (20 times higher than that for reversing AA).
- Plasma cAMP levels decrease during AA but rise during stress analgesia.
- The periaquaductal gray is essential for AA but not for stress analgesia.
- Dorsolateral spinal cord lesion eliminate AA but not stress analgesia.

Nevertheless, a note of caution is needed here. Some animal models of AA are indeed stressful to the animals, especially those done in the awake conscious state using strong stimulation of the needles. One such experiment involves the rat model used by Professor Han of Beijing Medical University which has been recently challenged by Professor Mayer of the University of Virginia [16b–d].

2.1.3 Evidence for Midbrain Monoamines and Acupuncture Analgesia

There are numerous papers implicating the midbrain monoamines in AA (especially serotonin and norepinephrine). As the raphe magnus in the brainstem contains most of the serotonin cells in the brain, lesions which destroy these cells (or their axons in the DLT) would presumably impair AA if serotonin were involved (such lesions also abolish morphine analgesia, which is mediated by descending inhibition via the raphe-DLT-serotonin system) [9]. Numerous experiments show that lesions to this system in animals block AA [32, 45a, 83, 100a, 119, 171, 215]. Moreover, antagonistic drugs which block serotonin receptors, block AA in mice [32, 173]. In the above tests of the serotonin-AA hypothesis, the drugs were given systemically (usually i.p.). Local microinjection studies, however, produced surprising results, suggesting that the descending serotonin-DLT inhibitory system may not be as important as the raphe projections to the forebrain: intrathecal injections of serotonin antagonists over the spinal cord produced no blockade of AA in rats [136], while lesions of the ascending raphe tracts caused a selective decrease of cerebral serotonin and a correlated decrease of AA in the rat [66].

Microinjection of serotonin antagonists into the various brain regions confirmed the importance of ascending serotonin pathways; AA was blocked by injections into the limbic system and the midbrain PAG [66]. Enhancement of AA was observed in mice [32] and rats [66] when serotonin was increased by giving 5HTP (a precursor) systemically or intracerebroventricularly [66], the latter route being more effective than the intrathecal route. Measurement of 5HT and its metabolite 5-hydroxyindole-acetic acid (5HIAA) in the brain and spinal cord of rats during AA showed increased synthesis and utilization of 5HT [191a, 223c]. The importance of serotonin in AA has also been confirmed clinically in patients using the serotonin uptake blocker clomipramine, where AA was potentiated in a double-blind study [223b].

All this leaves us with the questions: why does a lesion of the DLT in the spinal cord inhibit AA [171] if spinal cord serotonin does not mediate AA effects? Does the DLT contain other transmitters which mediate AA? Mayer and Watkins suggest that a synergism between descending serotonin and norepinephrine is the possible answer [115]. Indeed, Hammond [65] showed that combined intrathecal antagonists (for serotonin and for norepinephrine) produced the best antagonism of descending analgesia produced by brainstem stimulation. Perhaps this should be tried for AA (combined intrathecal antagonists should block AA more effectively than single antagonists).

There have been studies on the effects of norepinephrine (alone without serotonin) on AA. Intrathecal injection of a norepinephrine antagonist blocked AA, showing the importance of descending norepinephrine pathways [67]. Clearly the monoamine story needs more work. If synergism of descending serotonin and norepinephrine is important, then combined intrathecal blockers should be used in all future studies of monoamines in AA. The relative roles of the ascending and descending tracts need to be clarified.

In conclusion, there is no doubt that the monoamines (serotonin and norepinephrine) play a role in AA. Serotonin projections from the raphe to higher centers may mediate AA. Descending projections to the spinal cord (via DLT) may work in synergism with descending norepinephrine effects to block pain transmission in the spinal cord.

2.1.4 Evidence for Pituitary Hypothalamic System and Acupuncture Analgesia

The third possible center mediating low-frequency endorphin analgesia is the pituitary-hypothalamic system. The arcuate nucleus of the ventromedial hypothalamus plus the pituitary gland contain all the β-endorphin cells in the brain [14]. As the arcuate cells have long axons, β-endorphin is found in other brain loci, but this all originates from the hypothalamic cells [203]. The arcuate cells can produce analgesia via these long axons (stimulating the midbrain PAG, for example). Lesions of the arcuate nucleus abolish AA in rats [167].

There is a good deal of confusion regarding the possible relationship of the pituitary (hormonal) β-endorphins to pain modulation. We have already mentioned the evidence (lesions and blood biochemistry studies) implicating pituitary endorphins in AA. Involvement of the pituitary in other forms of analgesia has also been studied. For example, stress-produced analgesia is at least partly mediated by pituitary β-endorphins [161]. Problems arise because pituitary ablation is a very unreliable technique: moreover, injection of the drug naloxone could have side effects. To make matters worse, in some species (e.g., rat) the blood-brain barrier for β-endorphin is quite tight [161], although mice, rabbits and man have less of a barrier [193]. Recently, a new route for the pituitary endorphins to reach the brain (bypassing the barrier) has been discovered [13, 124] in the hypothalamic pituitary portal system (reverse flow occurs). Perhaps the endorphins can reach the 3rd ventricles and, via the CSF, influence such structures as the PAG. Perhaps more important than the pituitary release of endorphins is the corelease of ACTH which occurs during AA [109, 113, 129] because this stimulates the adrenals to raise blood cortisol levels after AA [16, 35, 94, 99]. Sham acupuncture does not raise blood cortisol levels [35, 94] thus ruling out stress as the cause of cortisol release. It is tempting to speculate that this cortisol mediates the treatment effects of acupuncture in arthritis, effects which seem to go beyond analgesia [33]. Similarly asthma might be helped by cortisol release [12, 183, 185].

2.1.5 Conclusions

In conclusion, the evidence for the mediation of AA by endorphins is very strong, while that for the involvement of monoamines needs more work to verify the possible synergism of serotonin and norepinephrine. Moreover, the circuits depicted in Figs. 1 and 2 are quite well established, although there is some uncertainty about the role of the pituitary.

2.2 Acupuncture Analgesia for Chronic Pain

This section reaches two important conclusions. First, AA is very effective in treating chronic pain, helping from 55% to 85% of patients, which compares favorably with the effects of potent drugs (e. g., morphine helps in 70% of cases) [11]. Second, AA is more effective than placebo, indicating a real physical effect. There have been three recent reviews [96, 160, 197].

These conclusions are based on evidence collected in three classes of studies (all studies have been omitted in which fewer than two treatment sessions were given to each patient):

Class A studies in which there was no control group for comparison with the acupuncture group or in which there was a control group in which the subjects received no treatment whatsoever.

Class B studies in which there was a control group receiving percutaneous acupuncture but at the wrong location (called sham acupuncture). The sham-acupuncture group was compared with a group that received true acupuncture.

Class C studies using a placebo control group (usually a disconnected TENS device, or acupuncture needles taped to the skin) and in which this group was compared with the group receiving true acupuncture. It is important to note that needles were not inserted percutaneously in the control group for class C studies, and hence this is not considered to be sham acupuncture.

In classes B and C the experiments were usually single blind (the patient did not know about the sham or placebo but the therapist did know). We will show below that the quality of the experiments, in descending order, is class C, class B, class A. Initially it was thought that class B studies were similar in quality to those of class C; it was hoped that sham acupuncture was a good control for placebo effects, and thus many studies were based on this approach [160, 197]. Unfortunately, experience has since shown that sham acupuncture (needles inserted in wrong locations in class B) helps about 33%–50% of chronic pain patients [160, 197], while placebo in class C helps only 30%–35% of patients [160, 197] (as mentioned above "true" acupuncture helps 55%–85% of patients) [160, 197]. In the review by Lewith and Machin [96] it was argued convincingly that the statistical problems inherent in class B experiments, in which one group shows a 40% success rate (sham acupuncture) and another one shows a 70% success rate (true acupuncture), make the burden of proof unrealistic, requiring at least 122 patients in the study to find a difference between the two groups.

As stated above, placebo benefits only 30%–35% of patients with chronic pain. Hence the burden of proof is more realistic for class C experiments: to compare 30% in placebo controls with 70% in true acupuncture requires only 70 patients (35 per group, 70 total). Hence, it is not surprising that all class C experiments showed significant differences between treated and controls [107, 141, 160 a], while 6 out of 11 class B experiments did not ([48, 57, 58, 222] but see [43 b, 64 a, 73, 114, 197 b]). We can conclude from class C studies that acupuncture helps 55%–85% of chronic pain patients, and this is significantly better than placebo controls, only 30%–35% of whom have been helped [107, 141]. In class B, despite the failures to observe significant differences between sham and true acupuncture groups, it could be that the 33%–50% success rates observed with sham acupuncture were not entirely placebo effects as these rates were in excess of the 30%–35% generally seen in placebo studies. Moreover, the class B results suggest (but do not prove) that acupuncture points may not be very specific in their ability to produce analgesia. To avoid statistical problems, class B studies with larger sample sizes (122 patients) are needed, for thorough testing of the specificity of acupuncture points versus sham points for treatment of chronic pain.

Normally we would completely ignore class A experiments, as they are poorly controlled studies. Perhaps this is too severe, as many of these studies showed the 55%–85% success rate [26, 27, 42, 43, 84, 89, 93, 95, 155, 178, 223] that is now known from class C experiments to be far above the placebo level of 30%–35%. Strictly speaking, comparison across experiments is not permissible, but one cannot help but be impressed with the consistency of all the results in each of classes A, B and C.

In addition to the three classes of studies outlined above, there have been several experiments in which the acupuncture group was compared with a group receiving standard treatments for chronic pain. These studies suffered from the same problems as class B experiments (placing too strong a burden of proof on the small sample size). Nevertheless, several of these studies did show that AA outperformed the standard medical treatment [62, 101, 103, 180], while others [2, 99 a–c] showed no differences between AA and conventional therapies (the latter result may be due to a type II error because of small sample size). However, even if the analgesic effects of acupuncture and of a chemical analgesic are equivalent, this is also a victory for AA, given the many side effects of analgesic drugs (in comparison with drugs AA has very few side effects; see Chap. 5). In two additional studies in which acupuncture was compared with TENS, acupuncture was slightly more effective, but the differences were not statistically significant [52, 90] because of a type II error due to small sample size. A major flaw in many class A, B and C clinical trials was the failure to elicit De Qi sensations. When deliberate efforts were made to activate type III fibers and produce De Qi the success rate was 85%–90% even after 4–8 months follow-up [33].

A recent meta-analysis of 14 different controlled studies, used a new statistical method which permitted the authors to pool data from many diverse experimental designs: this meta-analysis showed statistical significance in favour of acupuncture over the control groups [133 b].

However, a more recent meta-analysis based on 51 controlled clinical studies concluded that "the efficacy of acupuncture in the treatment of chronic pain remains doubtful" [187 b]. It is unfortunate that the latter paper, which carefully listed "criteria" for paper selection, failed to mention De Qi, intensity of stimulation, or number of treatment sessions as important factors. In statistics there is a well-known cliché: "garbage-in, garbage-out." In meta-analysis this cliché is most relevant! By including papers in which negative results were obtained from improper acupuncture, the positive results of other studies were cancelled out [187 b].

In conclusion, we see that AA works better than placebo (class C) for most pains (except neuralgias or migraines) [44, 97] and helps 55%–85% of patients, which is a remarkable efficacy rate; morphine only helps 70% of patients with chronic pain [11]. If AA is better than or equal to conventional methods, and if AA is safer than drugs, then AA should become the method of choice for treating certain chronic pains. Further studies in class C would make these conclusions even more convincing. Experiments in class B and A are poorly designed, but the success rate of AA in them seems too high to be merely a placebo effect. Future studies should attempt to optimize De Qi sensations to see whether a higher success rate can be achieved.

Finally a comment on the nature of placebo is relevant here. The half-life of AA is 15–17 min in man and 7–13 min in rabbits [68a, b]. This cannot be explained by placebo, which is much more transient: these long time courses are typical of morphine effects, and not of placebo. Another major difference between acupuncture and placebo effect is the fact that repeated acupuncture treatments potentiate this effect, while repeated placebos become less and less effective each time [87a].

2.3 Drug Addiction

Wen, a well-known Hong Kong neurosurgeon, discovered fortuitously that EA produced relief of the withdrawal symptoms of opium addiction. He found this when he gave acupuncture for postsurgical pain to his patients, some of whom turned out to be closet opium addicts. In his first paper on this subject he reported that prolonged daily ear acupuncture treatments for 8 days helped patients withdraw from opium [205], but in a later paper he reported that a more rapid and effective method of treatment was to combine the antagonist naloxone with EA given for 30 min a day for 3 days [204]. Wen did not claim a cure: "The treatment was not a cure because craving for the drug, even without any abstinence symptoms, still persisted in these patients. Therefore it should be said that a patient has been detoxified but that he still needs rehabilitation, especially on the psychosocial side" [204].

24

Other studies have shown lower success rates, perhaps due to motivation problems and high dropout rates before a course of treatment was completed [110]. Other researchers have shown good initial results. Excluding papers in acupuncture journals, we counted six successful replications of Wen's work [87, 102, 135, 163, 170, 201 d]. In one study [170] involving patients addicted to analgesics, 12 out of 14 patients were successfully withdrawn [170] using ear points for 60 min a day.

Several authors speculated that endorphin release mediated this effect [36, 127, 170, 207, 208, 209]. Perhaps the most impressive study of all was recently reported by Bullock, who treated chronic alcoholics with ear acupuncture; of 50 patients 25 received three needles in true ear points, and 25 received three sham needles in wrong ear points. Despite being offered liquor ad. lib., 42% of alcoholics remained alcohol free for 3 months, and an additional 28% drank much less (for a total of 70% success) when given true acupuncture [17 b]. Hence acupuncture reduced craving and did not merely suppress withdrawal. Sham had no effect. Replications are needed for this important finding. Bullock et al. [17 c] have recently repeated this finding in 80 patients with similar results; other studies are currently under way in several other centers.

At this point we should mention a recent meta-analysis of 22 studies of the effect of acupuncture on addiction. Their conclusion was that "claims that acupuncture is efficacious as a therapy for these addictions are thus not supported by results from sound clinical research" [187 a]. The "garbage-in, garbage-out" criticism which was raised previously for meta-analysis of chronic pain studies applies here as well. Should 20 bad studies negate the two good studies? Why were factors such as combined acupuncture plus intense psychotherapy not used as a prerequisite for inclusion in the meta-analysis? More work is needed.

Since this meta-analysis was performed there has been intense interest by National Institute of Drug Abuse (NIDA) in the USA to fund controlled clinical trials of acupuncture for addiction. This has arisen because of a worldwide surge in the use of acupuncture to treat opium and cocaine addictions. Based on the highly successful treatment program developed by Smith at New York City's Lincoln Hospital during the 1970s [175 a], over 400 treatment centers have been established worldwide [16f]. The strategy combines ear acupuncture for 30 min a day, with group psychotherapy. Several law enforcement agencies in the USA give addicts the choice of jail or acupuncture!

2.4 Nerve Regeneration, Cardiovascular, Antiemetic and Urogenital Effects of Acupuncture

These topics are all covered under one heading because very little controlled research has been done in any of these areas.

Nerve regeneration in humans has not been subjected to proper double-blind clinical studies. In China there have been anecdotal reports of over 100000 cases of Bell's palsy (paralysis of the 7th nerve) treated with acupuncture, with a success rate of 92%. However, Bell's palsy shows spontaneous remission in over 80% of cases, so we cannot draw any conclusions without a placebo control group. In laboratory experiments, my group showed that EA markedly enhanced motor-nerve regeneration and sensory nerve sprouting in adult rats after sciatic nerve injury [118, 145, 154]. Naeser et al. recently completed studies at Boston Veterans Hospital to study the effect of acupuncture on patients with cerebrovascular accidents, with positive results [126a–c].

Many cardiovascular experiments have been done on animals. In one elegant experiment Yao et al. [219] used acupuncturelike stimulation of the sciatic nerve to lower blood pressure for prolonged periods in awake, spontaneously hypertensive rats. This was replicated in another recent study [79]. These effects were naloxone reversible and had a serotonin component [219] much like AA. In another study Thoren showed that prolonged "jogging" in spontaneously hypertensive rats produced exactly the same effects as acupuncture (jogging produced analgesia and lowered blood pressure via serotonin and endorphin mechanisms), suggesting that type III muscle afferents may function normally to induce analgesia during severe exercise [189]. (Incidentally, the jogger's high and analgesia from running are both antagonized by naloxone in humans.) Evolution did not create type III muscle afferents for acupuncturists!

Anesthetized dogs stimulated at Du 26 (the upper lip) show a rise in blood pressure which is not antagonized by naloxone [91]. Moreover, in hemorrhagic shock in dogs, stimulation of this point helps to restore the blood pressure by increasing cardiac output [41]. The same authors working with dogs observed that the lowering of cardiac output that could be obtained by stimulating St. 36 was blocked by atropine, suggesting a parasympathetic effect. Recent studies in anesthetized cats and rats showed that low-intensity stimulation lowered the secretion of catecholamines from the adrenal medulla, while high-intensity activation of peripheral nerves increased secretion. In turn, these lowered secretions reduced blood pressure, while elevated secretions increased blood pressure [6]. Recent studies by Ernst and Lee indicate that acupuncture of Li. 4 and St. 36 causes cutaneous vasodilatation in normal human subjects as shown by elegant thermography studies [49 a, b]. Finally recent research showed that manual and electroacupuncture enhanced survival of musculocutaneous flaps by preventing local ischemia [81 a, b].

In a recent series of papers the effectiveness of treating nausea has been clearly demonstrated using Pe. 6 Neiguan, the median nerve in the lower forearm. In 10 out of the 12 papers published, the treatment was very effective. Of these ten successful studies, six used a placebo control group [8 a, 46 a–d, 78 a], two had a no treatment control group [38 a, 79 a], and two had a drug treatment control group [1 a, 57 a]. Acupuncture was found to be more effective than the placebo or no treatment controls, and was equally effective to the drug groups. In the ten successful papers a variety of stimulations of Pe. 6 were used: acupressure, manual twirling, or electroacupuncture were all equally effective. Of these ten studies, six were for postoperative nausea [8 a, 38 a, 46 a, 46 c, 57 a, 78 a], two were for morning sickness of pregnancy [46 d, 79 a], and two were for nausea after cancer chemotherapy [1 a, 46 b]. The one failed experiment used acupressure to treat laboratory induced nausea. [17 a]. All together there is a critical mass of data supporting the effectiveness of acupuncture in treating nausea. Another failed experiment gave acupuncture at the wrong time: after induction of anesthesia and before surgery [220a]. These results with acupressure at Pe. 6 have been less powerful in serious cases of vomiting [95a, 201a] but quite effective for milder problems such as morning sickness of pregnancy [43a]. Given the enormous danger of drug therapy in the pregnant woman, acupressure would be preferable to drugs for treatment of morning sickness. However the mechanism of action remains obscure. Do sensory inputs from the median nerve somehow reach the area postrema of the brainstem to block nausea? Anesthetic blockade of the median nerve with lidocaine was shown to block these effects [46f]. Electrophysiology could perhaps solve this important problem.

There have been a few recent clinical papers suggesting the usefulness of acupuncture in treatment of urogenital problems. In one study real acupuncture was superior to needling of sham points in treating dysmenorrhea [75b]. In another two studies, bladder problems were improved [20a, 141a] but only one of these two trials used a sham control. In the fourth urogenital study, TENS was used at acupoints to determine its effectiveness on uterine contractions in pregnancies past the due-date. For sham TENS, a control group had a disconnected device. Real treatments produced a significantly greater increase in strength and frequency of uterine contractions than the sham group [47a]. Obviously, more work is needed to confirm these urogenital effects of acupuncture.

2.5 Acupuncture Points (Do They Really Exist?)

The question of the existence of acupuncture points has been explored in several ways:

1. By comparing the effects of needling at true points versus sham points
2. By studying the unique anatomical structures at acupoints
3. By studying the electrical properties of skin at acupoints
4. By studying the nerves being activated by acupuncture at acupoints

2.5.1 Does Needling at True Points Work Better Than Needling at Sham Points?

Several experimenters have shown, for acute laboratory-induced pain in human subjects, that needling of true points produces marked analgesia while needling of sham points produces very weak effects [16e, 22, 179]. These results were clear-cut because effects elicited by sham-point stimulation are nonexistent in acute laboratory pain (placebo pills also have poor efficacy in acute pain, causing analgesia in only 3% of cases). In contrast to these clearcut results, the work on chronic pain patients has been less convincing. As mentioned in Section 2.2, placebo analgesia in chronic pain has a strong effect, working in 30%–35% of patients. Moreover, needling in sham points seems to work in about 33%–50% of patients, while true points are effective in about 55%–85% of cases [197]. Therefore, to show statistical significance in the differences between sham-point needling and true-point needling requires huge numbers of patients (at least 122 per study), and experiments that would allow definitive conclusions have not yet been done [197] (see Sect. 2.2). It is puzzling that sham acupuncture works in 33%–50% of patients with chronic pain, while not working at all in acute laboratory-induced pain. Because of these problems the specificity of acupoints has only been shown in acute pain studies in humans but has yet to be properly studied in patients with chronic pain, where the number of patients studied has never exceeded the required statistical minimum of 122.

In animal studies in mouse [149], cat [19, 56], horse [35], rat [182, 188], and rabbit [55, 99], many researchers have shown that true acupuncture works better than sham needling in acute pain studies. These results are consistent with the research on acute pain in humans. It is important in such studies to use mild stimulation in awake animals to avoid inducing stress; strong stimulation of sham sites could cause stress-induced analgesia [144]. Stress analgesia is a well-documented phenomenon [108] and is after mediated by endorphins. If the stimulation used is very strong, animals are highly stressed by both true- and sham-point needling.

Hence numerous studies on *acute* pain in animals and humans clearly demonstrate that AA from needling true points is far superior to AA from needling sham points. However, more studies are needed on *chronic* pain to see whether true points are more effective than sham points.

2.5.2 Are There Unique Anatomical Structures at Acupuncture Points?

Despite several histological studies of the skin and subcutaneous structures under acupoints, no unique structures have been found. However, several authors [62, 123] have made the astute observation that the majority of acupuncture points coincide with trigger points. For example, Melzack et al. found that 71% of acupuncture points correspond to trigger points [123]. This suggests that needles activate the sensory nerves which arise in muscles. This agrees with findings that stimulation of muscle afferents is important for producing analgesia [37, 104, 201]. The work of Travell on trigger points, beginning in 1952 [190] and culminating in a large book published in 1983 [191], shows that there are small hypersensitive loci in the myofascial structures, which when touched or probed give rise to a larger area of pain in an adjacent or distant (referred) area. She observed that "dry needling" (with needles containing no drugs) of these trigger points produced pain relief. When sites are tender the Chinese call them Ah Shi points, and needling of them is recommended. Often trigger points can be found outside muscle bellies, in skin, scars, tendons, joint capsules, ligaments and periosteum [191]. Travell stresses the importance of precise needling of trigger points as missing the tense knotted muscle fiber could aggravate the problem by causing spasms. Similarly, strong electrical stimulation should be avoided. Thus mild stimulation with needles inserted directly into trigger points is recommended [191]. Commonest trigger points are located on (or near) the following acupoints: Sl.10–13, 15; SJ.13, 14; UB.12–17, 28, 29, 36–41, 48, 49; and GB.27–30, 50. Although the cause of trigger point tenderness is unknown, one possibility is that poor inactivation of calcium by muscle sarcoplasmic reticulum causes calcium to cross-link the actin and myosin with ensuing permanent contracture. How needling rectifies this problem, however, is unclear [191].

In a recent review on the subject of the anatomy of acupuncture points, Dung [47] listed ten structures which are found in the vicinity of acupoints (see especially numbers 5, 6, and 9 regarding trigger points). In decreasing order of importance, he found:

1. Large peripheral nerves. The larger the nerve, the better.
2. Nerves emerging from a deep to a more superficial location.
3. Cutaneous nerves emerging from deep fascia.
4. Nerves emerging from bone foramina.
5. Motor points of neuromuscular attachments: a neuromuscular attachment is the site where a nerve enters the muscle mass. This is not always the actual neuromuscular synapse, which may occur a few centimeters further along the nerve and after it has divided into smaller branches. The pathophysiological significance of this neuromuscular attachment is unknown. Travell emphasises that many authors have used "motor point" interchangeably with "trigger point," but they are not at the same location in most cases [191].
6. Blood vessels in the vicinity of neuromuscular attachments.
7. Along a nerve which is composed of fibers of varying sizes (diameters). This is more likely on muscular nerves than on cutaneous nerves.
8. Bifurcation point of peripheral nerve.
9. Ligaments (muscle tendons, joint capsules, fascial sheets, collateral ligaments), as they are rich in nerve endings.
10. Suture lines of the skull.

It is obvious from this list that no particular structure dominates at acupuncture points. Perhaps the major correlate is the presence of nerves, be they in large nerve bundles (items 1–8) or nerve endings (items 9 and 10).

A recent report by Heine revealed that 80% of acupoints correlate with perforations in the superficial fascia of cadavers. Through these holes, a cutaneous nerve vessel bundle penetrates to the skin. If replicated, this finding could be the morphological basis for acupoints [75 a].

The abolition of AA by injection of local anesthetics into an acupoint before stimulation begins [37, 151] strongly suggests that nerves are important for this phenomenon (see Sect. 2.5.4). However, we should not rule out other mechanisms to explain effects of acupuncture in immunological, allergic, and other non-AA phenomena. One can speculate on the possible release of arachidonic acid from lesioned membranes during needling, giving rise to leukotrienes and prostaglandins, which could affect immunity. Also, currents of injury (electric currents generated from a hole in the skin) might be important for nerve regeneration (see Sect. 2.5.3). Do local anesthetics prevent all acupuncture effects, as they do for AA? It would be easy to find out, but few experiments have been done on non-analgesic effects. Recent evidence suggests the existence of channels which may correlate with meridians. Vernejoul et al. [196 a] injected subcutaneously (to a depth of 4 mm) a radioactive isotope into 130 humans, using technetium-99 in sodium pertechnetate in a volume of 0.05 ml. They compared migration of the isotope (using a gamma camera) after injection into acupoints with injection into non-acupoints. They claimed that vertical lines of migration were seen only from acupoints. These extended as far as 30 cm within 5 min and resembled meridian lines in their distribution. Moreover the migration velocity was altered under pathological conditions. From the photographs in the papers, however, it was difficult to draw conclusions. Also, one must rule out lymphatic drainage. Several recent reports have favored venous drainage as the explanation for this isotope migration raising serious doubts about this method for studying meridians [90 a, 174 a, 215 a, 216 a]. Replications by other laboratories are definitely needed before conclusions can be drawn from this controversial research.

2.5.3 Do Acupuncture Points Have Unique Physiological Features?

There have been a number of reports that the skin resistance (impedance) over acupuncture points is lower than that of surrounding skin [10, 18], but this result has been attributed to pressure artifacts from electrodes [117, 131, 192]. Normally dry skin has a DC resistance in the order of 200000–2 million ohms. At acupuncture points this is down to 50000 ohms in the studies claiming unique properties of acupoints. These observations have led to the marketing of "point finders," pencil-shaped metal-tipped probes attached by wires to an ohmmeter. The circuit is completed by a second electrode in a hand-held metal cylinder (with large skin contact on the sweaty palm and hence with a low resistance in the order of 1000 ohms). The point finder generally measures DC resistance based on Ohm's law ($E = IR$): a constant voltage is applied to the wires, and the resultant current (I) is measured, from which resistance (R) is instantly computed. This can be read out on a meter directly or a Wheatstone bridge. Most devices produce a beeping tone whose frequency (or intensity) is proportional to the resistance being measured. This allows the clinician to move the roving pencil probe around the body surface while listening to the tones. Anecdotal reports suggest that these devices work best in certain regions (e.g., hands, face, ears) in which acupuncture points and low resistance often coincide (but see [121] for negative results on the ear). It is further claimed that during disease of particular organs the resistances at acupoints are abnormally low (even lower than the usual low resistance at acupoints; but see [121]). Indeed, the Japanese (Ryodoraku) method of measuring the acupoint skin resistance on the body has been in widespread use in Japan since it was introduced by Nakatani in 1950 [128], while Nogier and the French school [130] have made observations at ear acupoints (but see also [121]). In Germany, the Voll machine has concentrated on another skin electrical phenomenon, whereby the initial peak resistance reading is ignored while the capacitative "fall-back" of the reading to a steady-state (higher resistance) value is considered diagnostic. In the USSR, Gaikin developed the toboscope as a point finder, which was shown at the World Fair in Montreal in 1967. This was further developed by Nechushkin in the 1970's.

There have been two careful experiments to validate the claims of ear "point finders" [121, 133]. Oleson et al. [133] took 40 patients and in an "blind" design compared diagnoses made by using a point finder (9 V DC, 50 µA) on the ear with diagnoses made on the same patients by means of a Western medical work-up. The researchers were blind as to the Western diagnosis, to ensure that no clues were available to them. Amazingly, the correlation between ear diagnosis and Western diagnosis was 72.5%, which was highly significant [133]. Recently, Melzack and Katz [121] could find no difference in conductance between acupuncture points and nearby control points in patients with chronic pain [121] when they measured skin resistances in the ear. Unfortunately, neither Ryodoraku nor the Voll machine has been validated by similar controlled studies. Moreover, the further claims for the Voll machine that homeopathic remedies placed in parallel with the measuring wires can modify the readings, and thereby be used to select appropriate treatments for the diagnosed ailment, have never been scientifically tested [83a].

Until recently we were quite sceptical of the entire skin resistance phenomenon. This was because the measurements were not made in accordance with established biophysical practice. Neither published reports [10, 18, 157, 158] nor clinical anecdotal observations had been based on properly conducted studies, as pointed out by others [18, 117, 131, 192]. Recently we have improved the methodology. To avoid electrochemical potentials Ag/AgCl electrodes were used with a salt bridge; to avoid polarization from DC currents biphasic pulses were used; to avoid electrical damage to skin small (microampere) currents were applied; to avoid mechanical injury of the skin springloaded probes were used; and to overcome skin moisture variations very small amounts of saline were supplied through a millipore filter from the salt bridge. When these precautions were taken a highly reliable technique was developed [174]. Preliminary results to date suggest that acupuncture points sometimes do have a lower impedance (resistance) than surrounding skin. Whether or not acupoints will turn out to have a lower skin resistance than surrounding skin, the point finders commercially available are very unreliable [174].

We have no idea what the physiological significance (if any) could be of low resistance at acupoints. It is known that sweating has a profound effect on skin resistance; this forms the basis of lie detector tests. Stress, which activates the sympathetics, causes sweating and a drop in skin resistance. In a preliminary study we have determined that sweating occurs uniformly over the skin surface (equally at acupoints and over the surrounding skin). Moreover, the ear lobe is practically devoid of sweat glands, yet resistance phenomena are claimed to occur there as well [133] (but see [121]). We have not yet validated the claims that there is a drop in resistance during disease; if this latter phenomenon proves to be true, the pathophysiological mechanism is unclear. Can sympathetics affect local sweating during disease? Why should this be localized to acupoints, when sweating normally appears to be diffusely organized? It is also unclear why, in normal people, the acupoint should have a low resistance. Could the presence of a large nerve, emerging from deep tissues to more superficial layers, induce skin changes?

Another finding at acupuncture points is the presence of a voltage source [10] (i.e., there is reported to be a potential difference between acupoints and the neighboring skin), with the points being 5 mV further in the positive direction than the non-points. Unfortunately (as mentioned above for resistance), most of these voltage measurements did not use state-of-the-art biophysical methodology. This is particularly unfortunate as electrochemical potential artifacts produced at the electrode-to-skin interface are large compared with the millivolts being generated by the body. Recently an outstanding study was published by Jaffe et al. [81], showing that the human skin has a resting potential across its epidermal layer of from 20 to 90 mV (outside negative, inside positive). This paper paid no attention to acupuncture points. Nevertheless, one can speculate that acupuncture points, having low resistance, tend to short-circuit this battery across the skin, and hence give rise to a source of current in a source-sink map of the skin. In other words, acupuncture points provide a path of least resistance for currents driven by the 20 to 90-mV resting potential which exists across the entire skin, and this is consistent with the 5 mV readings mentioned above [10].

An important measurement in the same paper by Jaffe et al. [81] showed that a lesion (a cut) in the skin produces a current of injury which is due to short-circuiting of the skin battery. Preliminary results [174] indicate that insertion of acupuncture needles into the skin might also produce a current of injury which has biological influences on the underlying tissues. Indeed, our team has recently reported that weak currents (only 1–10 µA) promote nerve growth in the leg of an adult rat when applied through acupuncture needles [118, 145, 147a, 154]. In China over 100000 patients with Bell's palsy of the 7th nerve have been reported (anecdotally) to benefit from EA and plain needling (see Sect. 2.4 above) [216]. Perhaps the current of injury caused by needling (and generated by the 20- to 90-mV resting potential across the intact skin) promotes nerve regeneration in these cases. It is important to note that nerves grown in cell cultures will grow branches toward the electrodes in a weak DC electric field [134]. Moreover, this growth is maximal in the direction of the negative pole [134]. The papers from our laboratory also show enhanced nerve growth towards the negative pole of the applied DC field [118, 145, 147a, 154]. Holes made by needles would also cause a negativity at the site of injury, due to the current of injury.

Regeneration of amputated amphibian limbs has been shown to be enhanced by applied electric fields (and currents), in the direction of the negative pole [15]. Although this has not been shown in adult mammals, there is indirect evidence of its effects in humans. If children suffer accidental amputation of the distal phalanx it will completely regenerate (with nail, fingerprint, etc.) provided the tissue is kept moist. The latter allows a current of injury which is negative distally and about 1 µA in amplitude [80].

DC fields and currents have also been implicated in bone healing, plant growth, embryology and spinal cord regeneration in paraplegic guinea pigs [132].

Preliminary studies on normal human volunteers in our laboratory indicate that needling the skin produces decrease of local skin resistance which lasts 1–2 days [174]. A simple calculation using Ohm's law suggests to us that a small hole created by an acupuncture needle can create a sufficient current of injury (10 µA) to be of possible benefit to tissue growth and regeneration [15, 145]. It should be noted that these tiny currents would not be sufficient to initiate nerve impulses, and hence the mechanisms shown in Figs. 1 and 2 would not be relevant here.

2.5.4 What Nerves Are Activated by Acupuncture?

Electrophysiological evidence (given below) indicates that stimulation of muscle afferent fibers (types II and III) produces De Qi sensations [201], which in turn send messages of the brain to release neurochemicals (endorphins, monoamines, cortisol). Perhaps acupoints are the loci of type II and III fibers.

In a recent review Omura emphasized the importance of eliciting strong muscle contractions to optimize AA; this, he says, requires low frequency EA to avoid tetanic contractions [133a]. Strong muscle contractions are elicited because the stimulus intensites required to activate the type III afferents fibers must be 5 to 10 times threshold for the muscle efferents (see Chap.7).

One of the earliest and most clear-cut papers on the subject was published by Chiang in 1973 [37]; in this paper he showed that the essential correlate of analgesia was a De Qi sensation: the feeling of numbness, fullness, and sometimes soreness [37]. By injecting procaine (2%) into the acupoints (LI.4 and LI.10) in humans he determined that subcutaneous injections did not block De Qi sensations, while intramuscular procaine abolished them. Moreover, whenever De Qi was blocked, so was AA. (Experiments have been done in animals [19, 55, 151] showing that procaine injections also abolish AA.) To rule out the role of circulating compounds released by acupuncture, he also repeated these experiments with a tourniquet on the arm: as the De Qi persisted, so did the AA. Another important finding recorded in Chiang's paper was the lack of target specificity: acupuncture of points in the arm produced equal AA in all parts of the body as measured by skin analgesia tests (he did not test the arm itself or he would have seen a stronger segmental effect there) [37]. Two other studies showed the same lack of target specificity in humans in acute laboratory-induced pain [100, 106]. This lack of target specificity is consistent with the mechanisms in Fig.2. It must be strongly emphasized here that the authors of the last two papers mentioned may have drawn the wrong conclusions from their otherwise excellent studies: they concluded that all the relief experienced was purely a placebo effect, since there was no targeting of the treatment effects to specific pain locations. Yet it is not possible that 60% of patients could have benefited from placebo: as stated previously, Beecher reports that in acute laboratory-induced pain, placebo only works in 3% of volunteers [11], and hence the 60% effect in the acute pain studies [106] could not have been mediated by placebo. Since they stimulated true acupoints they observed widespread AA effects. We interpret all these findings as follows: the acupoint maps are essential for localizing the sites where the best De Qi can be achieved (i.e., location of type II and III muscle afferents). In that sense, the points are specific. However, the further claim of traditional Chinese medicine, that the points are also target-specific, may not be true. The conclusion that point specificity is not total nonsense comes from the many studies on acute pain (both in humans and animals) in which sham acupuncture produces no analgesia. Here "sham" is used to mean placement of needles in nonacupoints (see Sect. 2.2). Remember that Lynn and Perl [106] placed needles in true acupoints, but they were merely inappropriate for the pain targets. Their points were not truly sham, in that they did not use nonacupoints. There have been numerous studies using proper sham acupuncture. In one human study acupuncturing the first dorsal interosseus muscle (LI.4) produced a rise in tooth pain threshold (using signal detection theory), while acupuncture of the fourth dorsal interosseus muscle (sham) produced no analgesia [22]. Another study of the pain threshold of the neck produced similar results [179]. Numerous animal studies have shown the same specificity: in mice [149], cats [19, 56], horses [35], rats [188], and rabbits [55, 99], the sham points showed no AA while real points gave AA. The most extensive series of experiments on sham acupuncture was performed by Takeshige et al. in Japan, on rats. Not only did this group find that non-acupuncture (sham) points failed to produce AA (in contrast to true points in the same animals), but they proceeded to find a plausible explanation [54, 77, 78, 86, 125, 142, 167, 181, 182, 182b, 182e, 195]. In a series of elegant experiments (far too complex to give in detail here) they mapped out an AA-inhibitory system in the brain which is activated by stimulation of nonacupoints: this system is activated from nonacupoints via nerves to the posterior hypothalamus, then to the lateral contromedian nucleus of the thalamus and finally to lateral PAG (where it inhibits the midbrain AA system). (For a review of this extensive research project, see [182].) Lesioning of this inhibitory system releases the suppressed AA, so that nonacupoints become effective in producing AA. Finally, Toda and Ichioka did an elegant experiment to show, in the rat, that lesioning of the ulnar nerve had no effect in blocking AA from LI.4 stimulation, but lesions of radial and median nerves abolished AA [188];

conversely, electrical stimulation of radial and median nerves produced AA but ulnar stimulation did not [188]. It appears that the ulnar nerve does not reach the analgesia sites of the brain. Recent experiments on nausea and vomiting showed that procaine into Pe. 6 blocked the acupuncture effect [46f].

This brings us to the most direct experiments of all: the recording of impulses from the nerves involved in producing AA. Pomeranz and Paley [151], recording from afferents from LI. 4 (first dorsal interosseus muscle) in mice, found that type II afferents were sufficient to produce AA. But they deliberately avoided activating pain fibers (types III and IV) in awake mice, to avoid causing stress analgesia. Similar results were reported by Toda and Ichioka, showing that type II afferents were sufficient for AA in the rat [188], as recruiting types III and IV did not augment the AA.

Experiments in monkeys, in which A-α and A-β fibers (i.e., types I and II) of the tibial nerve were electrically stimulated, resulted in only a slight inhibition of the pain responses of the spinothalamic pain tract [39a]. However, when the stimulus strength was increased to a level which excited A-δ (type III) fibers, a powerful inhibition was observed [39a]. Moreover, it should be emphasized that increasing the stimulus strength to excite C-fibers (type IV) is not necessary as it causes unbearable pain in conscious patients.

In a recent paper, Lu [104] showed that types II and III afferents were important in rabbits and cats for AA: dilute procaine (0.1%) blocked type IV fibers and had no effect on AA, while ischemic blockade (or anodal blockade) of types II and III fibers abolished AA. Thus, types II and III mediate AA in these two species (all blockades were verified with direct electrical recordings from the blockade nerves).

Perhaps the best experiment of all was recently done on humans with direct microelectrode recordings from single fibers in the median nerve while acupuncture was performed distally [201]. When De Qi was achieved the following was observed: type II muscle afferents produced numbness, type III gave sensations of heaviness, distension and aching and type IV (unmyelinated fibers), soreness. As soreness is an uncommon aspect of De Qi, we must conclude that the main components of De Qi are carried by types II and III afferents (small myelinated afferents from muscle).

A recent study of De Qi on 65 human volunteers supports the existence of theses sensations with needling. However they also reported a confusing finding in the same paper: it seems that sham needling at non-points produces as much De Qi as elicited from true classical acupoints [197 a]. More research is needed to confirm this paradox. If true then acupoints may not be site specific after all for AA if indeed AA is always elicited by De Qi. Perhaps this could explain the moderate success rate for AA achieved in some studies from sham AA. Unfortunately as mentioned above, very few studies discuss the De Qi aspect of the parameters of treatment which were used.

Finally, mention should be made of the sensation sometimes felt by the acupuncturist: the "grab" of the needle by the muscle when proper De Qi is achieved. Recordings of electromyograms around acupoints during De Qi have shown pronounced muscle activation, accompanied by the therapist's noting the grab of the needle [5].

The practical importance of all this could be summarized as follows: for AA it is important to use strong stimulation to achieve De Qi sensations; the acupuncture maps are specific in the sense of helping us find types II and III fibers needed to obtain De Qi. However, acupoints may not be target specific as claimed by meridian theory; the only target specificity occurs from segmental effects of Ah Shi (tender) point stimulation, in which there is an additional benefit from spinal segmental endorphins (see Fig. 2, cell 7), added to the total-body effect of midbrain and pituitary endorphins (see Fig. 2, cells 11 and 14). Thus, of the three acupuncture effects, local, meridian, and total body, we have evidence for local (Fig. 2, cell 7) and total body (Fig. 2, cells 11 and 14), but none (so far) for meridian effects.

References

1. Abrams SE, Reynolds AC, Cusick JF (1981) Failure of naloxone to reverse analgesia from TENS in patients with chronic pain. Anesth Analg 60: 81–84
1 a. Aglietti L, Roila F et al (1990) A pilot study of metoclopramide, dexamethasone, diphenhydramine and acupuncture in women treated with cisplatin. Cancer Chemother Pharmacol 26: 239–240

2. Ahonen E, Hakumaki M, et al (1983) Acupuncture and physiotherapy in the treatment of myogenic headache patients: pain relief and EMG activity. In: Bonica JJ (ed) Advances in pain research and therapy, vol 5. Raven, New York, pp 571–576

3. Andersson SA (1979) Pain control by sensory stimulation. In: Bonica JJ (ed) Advances in pain research and therapy, vol 3. Raven, New York, pp 561–585

4. Anonymous (Shanghai Inst Physiol) (1973) Acupuncture sensations and electromyogram of the needled point in patients with nervous diseases. [in Chinese] Chin Med J 53: 619–622

5. Anonymous (Shanghai Inst Physiol) (1973) Electromyographic activity produced locally by acupuncture manipulation. [in Chinese] Chin Med J 53: 532–535

6. Araki T, Ito K, Kurosawa M, Sato A (1984) Responses of adrenal sympathetic nerve activity and catecholamine secretion to cutaneous stimulation in anesthetized rats. Neuroscience 12: 289–299

6 a. Asamoto S, Takeshige C (1992) Activation of the satiety center by auricular acupuncture point stimulation. Brain Res Bull 29: 157–164

6 b. Ballegaard S, Pedersen F et al (1990) Effects of acupuncture in moderate stable angina pectoris: a controlled study. J Int Med 227: 25–30

7. Barber J, Mayer DJ (1977) Evaluation of the efficacy and neural mechanism of a hypnotic analgesia procedure in experimental and clinical dental pain. Pain 4: 41–48

8. Baron A, Shuster L et al (1975) Mouse strain variations of opiate receptors. Life Sci 17: 633–640

8 a. Barsoun G, Perry EP et al (1990) Postoperative nausea is relieved by acupressure. J R Soc Med 83: 66–89

9. Basbaum AI, Fields HL (1984) Endogenous pain control systems: brainstem spinal pathways and endorphin circuitry. Annu Rev Neurosci 7: 309–338

10. Becker RO, Reichmanis M et al (1976) Electrophysiological correlates of acupuncture points and meridians. Psychoenergetic Systems 1: 195–212

11. Beecher HK (1955) Placebo analgesia in human volunteers. J Am Med Assoc 159: 1602–1606

12. Berger D, Nolte D (1975) Acupuncture – has it a demonstrable bronchospasmolytic effect in bronchial asthma? Med Klin 70: P 1827–1830

13. Bergland RM, Page RB (1979) Pituitary–brain vascular relations. Science 204: 18–24

13 a. Bing Z, Villancuva L, Le Bars D (1990) Acupuncture and diffuse noxious inhibitory controls: naloxone-reversible depression of activities of trigeminal convergent neurons. Neuroscience 37: 809–818

13 b. Bing Z, Le Bars D et al (1991) Acupuncture-like stimulation induces a heterosegmental release of Met-enkephalin like material in the rat spinal cord. Pain 47: 71–77

14. Bloom F, Guillemin R et al (1978) Neurons containing β-endorphin in rat brain exist separately from those containing enkephalin: immunocytochemical studies. Proc Natl Acad Sci USA 75: 1591–1595
15. Borgens RB, Vanable JW, Jaffe LF (1979) Small artificial currents enhances *Xenopus* limb regeneration. J Exp Zool 207: 217–226
16. Bossut DF, Leshin LB, Stomberg MW (1983) Plasma cortisol and beta-endorphin in horses subjected to electro-acupuncture for cutaneous analgesia. Peptides 4: 501–507
16a. Bossut DF, et al (1986) Electroacupuncture-induced analgesia in sheep: measurement of cutaneous pain thresholds & plasma concentrations of prolactin & beta-endorphin immunoreactivity. Am J Vet Res 47: 669–676
16b. Bossut DF, Mayer DJ (1991) Electroacupuncture analgesia in naive rats: effects of brain stem and spinal cord lesions, and role of pituitary-andrenal axis. Brain Res 549: 52–58
16c. Bossut DF, Mayer DJ (1991) Electroacupuncture analgesia in rats: naltrexone antagonism is dependent on previous exposure. Brain Res 549: 47–51
16d. Bossut DF, Mayer DJ et al (1991) Electroacupuncture in rats: evidence for naloxone and naltrexone potentiation of analgesia. Brain Res 549: 36–46
16e. Brockhaus A, Elger CE (1990) Hypalgesic efficacy of acupuncture on experimental pain in men. Comparison of laser acupuncture and needle acupuncture. Pain 43: 181–185
16f. Brumbaugh AG (1992) Acupuncture: new perspectives in chemical dependency treatment. J Substance Abuse Treatment 10: 35–43
17. Boureau F, Willer JC, Yamaguchi Y (1979) Abolition par la naloxone de l'effect inhibiteur d'une stimulation électrique péripherique sur la composante tardive du reflex clignement. EEG Clin Neurophysiol 47: 322–328
17a. Bruce DG, Golding JF et al (1990) Acupressure and motion sickness. Aviat Space Environ Med 61: 351–365
17b. Bullock M, et al (1987) Acupuncture treatment of alcoholics. Alcoholism Clinical and Exp Res 11: 292–295
17c. Bullack ML et al (1989) Controlled trial fo acupuncture for severe recidivist alcoholism. Lancet 1: 1435–1439
18. Chan SHH (1984) What is being stimulated in acupuncture: evaluation of existence of a specific substrate. Neurosci Biobehav Rev 8: 25–33
19. Chan SHH, Fung SJ (1975) Suppression of polysynaptic reflex by electro-acupuncture and a possible underlying presynaptic mechanism in the spinal cord of the cat. Exp Neurol 48: 336–342
20. Chang HT (1980) Neurophysiological interpretation of acupuncture analgesia. Endeavour 4: 92–96
20a. Chang PL (1988) Urodynamic studies in acupuncture for women with frequency, urgency and dysuria. J Urol 140: 563–566

21. Chapman CR, Benedetti C (1977) Analgesia following TENS and its partial reversal by a narcotic antagonist. Life Sci 21: 1645–1648

22. Chapman CR, Chen AC, Bonica JJ (1977) Effects of intrasegmental electrical acupuncture on dental pain: evaluation by threshold estimation and sensory decision theory. Pain 3: 213–227

23. Chapman CR, Colpitts YM et al (1980) Evoked potential assessment of acupuncture analgesia: attempted reversal with naloxone. Pain 9: 183–197

24. Chapman R, Benedetti C et al (1983) Naloxone fails to reverse pain thresholds elevated by acupuncture: Acupuncture analgesia reconsidered. Pain 16: 13–31

25. Charlton G (1982) Naloxone reverses electroacupuncture analgesia in experimental dental pain. South Afr J Sci 78: 80–81

26. Chen GS (1977) Therapeutic effect of acupuncture for chronic pain. Am J Chin Med 5: 45–61

26a. Chen XH, Han JS (1992) All three types of opioid receptors in the spinal cord are important for 2/15 Hg electroacupuncture analgesia. Eur J Pharmacol 211: 203–210

26b. Chen XH, Han JS (1992) Analgesia induced by electroacupuncture of different frequencies is mediated by different types of opioid receptors: another cross-tolerance study. Behav Brain Res 47: 143–149

27. Cheng ACK (1975) The treatment of headaches employing acupuncture. Am J Chin Med 3: 181–185

28. Cheng R, Pomeranz B (1979) Correlation of genetic differences in endorphin systems with analgesic effects of D-amino acids in mice. Brain Res 177: 583–587

29. Cheng R, Pomeranz B (1979) Electroacupuncture analgesia is mediated by stereospecific opiate receptors and is reversed by antagonists of type 1 receptors. Life Sci 26: 631–639

30. Cheng R, Pomeranz B (1980) Electroacupuncture analgesia could be mediated by at least two pain-relieving mechanisms: endorphin and non-endorphin systems. Life Sci 25: 1957–1962

31. Cheng R, Pomeranz B (1980) A combined treatment with D-amino acids and electroacupuncture produces a greater anesthesia than either treatment alone: naloxone reverses these effects. Pain 8: 231–236

32. Cheng R, Pomeranz B (1981) Monoamineergic mechanisms of electroacupuncture analgesia. Brain Res 215: 77–92

33. Cheng R, Pomeranz B (1987) Electrotherapy of chronic musculoskeletal pain: comparison of electroacupuncture acupuncture-like TENS. Clin J Pain 2: 143–149

34. Cheng RS, Pomeranz B, Yu G (1979) Dexamethasone partially reduces and 2% saline treatment abolishes electroacupuncture analgesia: these findings implicate pituitary endorphins. Life Sci 24: 1481–1486

35. Cheng R, Pomeranz B et al (1980) Electroacupuncture elevates blood cortisol levels in naive horses: sham treatment has no effect. Int J Neurosci 10: 95–97

36. Cheng R, Pomeranz B, Yu G (1980) Electroacupuncture treatment of morphine dependent mice reduces signs of withdrawal without showing cross tolerance. Eur J Pharmacol 68: 477–481
37. Chiang CY, Chang CT et al (1973) Peripheral afferent pathway for acupuncture analgesia. Sci Sin 16: 210–217
38. Chou J, Tang J, Yang HY, Costa E (1984) Action of peptidase inhibitors on methionine5-enkephalin-arginine6-phenylalanine7 (YGGFMRF) and methionine5-enkephalin (YGGFM) metabolism and on electroacupuncture antinociception. J Pharmacol Exp Ther 230: 349–352
38 a. Christensen PA, Noreng M et al (1989) Electroacupuncture and postoperative pain. Br J Anaesth 62: 258–262
39. Chung JM, Willis WD et al (1983) Prolonged naloxone reversible inhibition of the flexion reflex in the cat. Pain 15: 35–53
39 a. Chung JM, Willis WD et al (1984) Factors influencing peripheral nerve stimulation produced inhibition of primate spinothalamic tract cells. Pain 19: 277–293
40. Clement-Jones V, Wen HL et al (1980) Increased beta-endorphin but not met-enkephalin levels in human CSF after acupuncture for recurrent pain. Lancet II: 946–949
40 a. Clement-Jones V, Wen HL et al (1979) Acupuncture in heroin addicts: changes in Met-enkephalin and beta endorphin in blood and CSF. Lancet II: 380–383
41. Clifford DH, Lee MO, Lee DC (1977) Cardiovascular effects of atropine on acupuncture, needling with electrostimulation at Tsu San Li (St36) in dogs. Am J Vet Res 38: 845–849
42. Coan RM, Wong G et al (1980) The acupuncture treatment of low back pain: a randomized controlled study. Am J Chin Med 8: 181–189
43. Coan RM, Wong G, Coan PL (1982) The acupuncture treatment of neck pain: a randomized controlled study. Am J Chin Med 9: 326–332
43 a. de Aloysio D, Penacchioni P (1992) Morning sickness control in early pregnancy by Neiguan Point acupressure. Obstet Gyn 80: 852–854
43 b. Deluze C, Bosia L et al (1992) Electroacupuncture in fibromyalgia: results of a controlled trial. BMJ 305: 1249–1252
44. Dowson DI, Lewith GT, Machin D (1985) The effects of acupuncture versus placebo in the treatment of headache. Pain 21: 35–42
45. Du HJ, Chao YF (1976) Localization of central structures involved in descending inhibitory effect of acupuncture on viscero-somatic discharges. Sci Sin 19: 137–148
45 a. Du HJ, Zimmerman M et al (1984) Inhibition of nociceptive neuronal responses in the cat's spinal dorsal horn by electrical stimulation and morphine microinjection in nucleus raphe magnus. Pain 19: 249–257
46. Du HJ, Chao YF (1979) Effect of destruction or stimulation of locus coeruleus on inhibition of viscero-somatic reflex activities. Acta Physiol Sin 31: 153–162

44

46a. Dundee JM, Chestnutt NM et al (1986) Traditional chinese acupuncture: a potentially useful antiemetic? Br Med J 233: 583–584

46b. Dundee JM, Ghaly RB et al (1989) Acupuncture prophylaxis of cancer chemotherapy induced sickness. J R Soc Med 82: 268–271

46c. Dundee JM, Ghaly RB et al (1989) Effect of stimulation of the P 6 antiemetic point on postoperative nausea and vomiting. Br J Anaesth 63: 612–618

46d. Dundee JM, Sourial FB et al (1989) P 6 acupressure reduces morning sickness. J R Soc Med 81: 456–457

46e. Dundee JW, Ghaly RG et al (1989) Effect of stimulation of the P 6 antiemetic point on postoperative nausea and vomiting. Br J Anesth 63: 612–618

46f. Dundee JW, Ghaly RG (1991) Local anesthesia blocks the antiemetic action of P 6 acupuncture. Clin Pharmacol Ther 50: 78–80

47. Dung HC (1984) Anatomical features contributing to the formation of acupuncture points. Am J Acupunct 12: 139–143

47a. Dunn PA, Rogers D, Halford K (1989) Transcutaneous electrical nerve stimulation at acupuncture points in the induction of uterine contractions. Obstet Gynecol 73: 286–290

48. Edelist G, Gross AE, Langer F (1976) Treatment of low back pain with acupuncture. Can Anaesth Soc J 23: 303–306

48a. Ekblom A, Hansson P (1991) Increased postoperative pain and consumption of analgesics following acupuncture. Pain 44: 241–247

48b. Ehrlich D, Haber P (1992) Influence of acupuncture on physical performance capacity and hemodynamic parameters. Int J Sports Med 13: 486–489

49. Ehrenpreis S (1985) Analgesic properties of enkephalinase inhibitors: animal and human studies. Prog Clin Biol Res 192: 363–370

49a. Ernst M, Lee MHM (1985) Sympathetic vasomotor charges induced by manual and electrical acupuncture of the Hoku point visualized by thermography. Pain 21: 25–33

49b. Ernst M, Lee MHM (1986) Sympathetic effects of manual and electrical acupuncture of the Tsousanli knee point: comparison with the Hoku hand point sympathetic effect. Exp Neurol 94: 1–10

50. Facchinetti F, Nappi G et al (1981) Primary headaches: reduced circulating beta-lipotropin and beta-endorphin levels with impaired reactivity to acupuncture. Cephalalgia 1: 195–201

51. Facchinetti F, Sandrini G et al (1984) Concomitant increase in nociceptive flexion reflex threshold and plasma opioids following transcutaneous nerve stimulation. Pain 19: 295–303

52. Fox EJ, Melzack R (1976) Transcutaneous electrical stimulation and acupuncture comparison of treatment for low back pain. Pain 2: 141–148

53. Fu TC, Halenda SP, Dewey WL (1980) The effect of hypophysectomy on acupuncture analgesia in the mouse. Brain Res 202: 33–39

54. Fujishita M, Hisamtsu M, Takeshige (1986) Difference between non-acupuncture point stimulation and AA after D-phenylalanine treat-

ment. [in Japanese (English abstract)] In: Takeshige C (ed) Studies on the mechanism of acupuncture analgesia based animal experiments. Showa University Press, Tokyo, p 638

55. Fung DTH, Chan SHH et al (1975) Electroacupuncture suppression of jaw depression reflex elicited by dentalgia in rabbits. Exp Neurol 47: 367–369

56. Fung SJ, Chan SHH (1976) Primary afferent depolarization evoked by electroacupuncture in the lumbar cord of the cat. Exp Neurol 52: 168–176

57. Gaw AC, Chang LW, Shaw LC (1975) Efficacy of acupuncture on osteoarthritic pain. N Engl J Med 21: 375–378

57 a. Ghaly RB, Fitzpatrick KT et al (1987) Antiemetic studies with traditional Chinese acupuncture. A comparison of manual needling with electrical stimulation & common antiemetics. Anaesthesia 42: 1108–1110

57 b. Gerhard I, Postneek K (1992) Auricular acupuncture in the treatment of female infertility. Gynecol Endocrin 6: 171–178

58. Ghia J, Mao W, Toomey T, Gregg J (1976) Acupuncture and chronic pain mechanisms. Pain 2: 285–299

59. Godfrey CM, Morgen P (1978) A controlled trial of the theory of acupuncture in musculoskeletal pain. J Rheumatol 5: 121–124

60. Goldstein A (1979) Endorphins and pain: a critical review. In: Beers RF (ed) Mechanisms of pain and analgesic compounds. Raven, New York, pp 249–262

61. Goldstein A, Hilgard EF (1975) Failure of the opiate antagonist naloxone to modify hypnotic analgesia. Proc Natl Acad Sci USA 72: 2041–2043

62. Gunn CC, Milbrandt WE et al (1980) Dry needling of muscle motor points for chronic low-back pain. Spine 5: 279–291

63. Ha H, Tan EC, Fukunaga H, Aochi O (1981) Naloxone reversal of acupuncture analgesia in the monkey. Exp Neurol 73: 298–303

64. Hachisu M, Takeshige C et al (1986) Abolishment of individual variation in effectiveness of acupuncture analgesia. [in Japanese (English abstract)] In: Takeshige C (ed) Studies on the mechanism of acupuncture analgesia based on animal experiments. Showa University Press, Tokyo, p 549

64 a. Haker E, Lundeberg T (1990) Acupuncture treatment of epicondylalgia: a comparative study of two acupuncture techniques. Clin J Pain 6: 221–226

65. Hammond DL (1985) Pharmacology of central pain modulating networks (biogenic amines and nonopioid analgesics). In: Fields H et al (eds) Advances in pain research and therapy. Raven, New York, pp 499–511

66. Han CS, Chou PH, Lu CC, Lu LH et al (1979) The role of central 5-HT in acupuncture analgesia. Sci Sin 22: 91–104

67. Han JS, Terenius L (1982) Neurochemical basis of acupuncture analgesia. Annu Rev Pharmacol Toxicol 22: 193–220

68. Han JS, Xie GX (1984) Dynorphin: important mediator for electroacupuncture analgesia in the spinal cord of the rabbit. Pain 18: 367–377

68a. Han JS, Zhou ZF, Xuan TY (1983) Acupuncture has analgesic effect in rabbits. Pain 15: 85–91

68b. Han JS (1986) Physiology and neurochemical basis of acupuncture analgesia. In: Cheng TO (ed) The international textbook of cardiology. Pergamon, New York, pp 1124–1132

68c. Han JS (1990) Differential release of enkephalin and dynorphin by low and high frequency electroacupuncture in the central nervous system. Acupuncture Sci Int J 1: 19–27

68d. Han JS, Terenius L et al (1991) Effect of low- and high-frequency TENS on met-enkephalin-arg-phe and dynorphin A immunoreactivity in human lumbar CSF. Pain 47: 295–298

68e. Han JS, Zhang RL (1993) Suppression of morphine abstinence syndrome by body electroacupuncture of different frequencies in rats. Drug Alcohol Dependence 31: 169–174

69. Han JS, Guan XM, Shu JM (1979) Study of central norepinephrine turnover rate during acupuncture analgesia in the rat. [in Chinese] Acta Physiol Sin 31: 11–19

70. Han JS, Li SJ, Tang J (1981) Tolerance to acupuncture and its cross tolerance to morphine. Neuropharmacology 20: 593–596

71. Han JS, Ding XZ, Fan SG (1985) Is cholecystokinin octapeptide (CCK-8) a candidate for endogenous antiopioid substrates? Neuropeptides 5: 399–402

71a. Han JS, Ding XZ, Fan SG (1986) Cholecystokinin octapeptide (DCK-8): antagonism to electroacupuncture analgesia and a possible role in electroacupuncture tolerance. Pain 27: 101–115

72. Han JS, Xie GX, Terenius L et al (1982) Enkephalin and beta endorphin as mediators of electroacupuncture analgesia in rabbits: an antiserum microinjection study. In: Costa E (ed) Regulatory peptides: from molecular biology to function. Raven, New York, pp 369–377

73. Hansen PE, Hansen JH (1983) Acupuncture treatment of chronic facial pain: a controlled cross-over trial. Headache 23: 66–69

73a. Hardebo JE, Ekman R, Eriksson M (1989) Low CSF Met-enkephalin levels in cluster headache are elevated by acupuncture. Headache 29: 494–497

74. Hayes R, Price DD, Dubner R (1977) Naloxone antagonism as evidence for narcotic mechanisms. Science 196: 600

74a. He L (1987) Involvement of endogenous opioid peptides in acupuncture analgesia. Pain 31: 99–121

74b. He L, Lu R, Zhuang S et al (1985) Possible involvement of opioid peptides of caudate nucleus in acupuncture analgesia. Pain 23: 83–93

75. He LF, Doug WQ, Wang MZ (1991) Effects of iontophoretic etorphine, naloxone and electroacupuncture on nociceptive responses from thalamic neurones in rabbits. Pain 44: 89–95

47

75 a. Heine H (1988) Akupunkturtherapie – Perforationen der oberflächlichen Körperfaszie durch kutane Gefäß-Nervenbündel. therapeutikon 4: 238–244

75 b. Helms JM (1987) Acupuncture for the management of primary dysmenorrhea. Obstet Gynecol 69: 51–56

76. Herget HF, LÁllemand H et al (1976) Combined acupuncture analgesia and controlled respiration. A new modified method of anesthesia in open heart surgery. Anaesthesist 25: 223–230

77. Hishida F, Takeshige C et al (1986) Differentiation of acupuncture point and non-acupuncture point explored by evoked potential of the central nervous system and its correlation with analgesia inhibitory system. [in Japanese (English abstract)] In: Takeshige C (ed) Studies on the mechanism of acupuncture analgesia based on animal experiments. Showa University Press, Tokyo, p 43

78. Hishida F, Takeshige C et al (1986) Effects of D-phenylalanine on individal variation of analgesia and on analgesia inhibitory system in their separated experimental procedures. [in Japanese (English abstract)] In: Takeshige C (ed) Studies on the mechanism of acupuncture analgesia based on animal experiments. Showa University Press, Tokyo, p 51

78 a. Ho RT, Jawan B (1990) Electroacupuncture and postoperative emesis. Anaesthesia 45: 327–329

78 b. Ho UK, Hen HL (1989) Opioid-like activity in the cerebrospinal fluid of pain patients treated by electroacupuncture. Neuropharmacology 28: 961–966

79. Hoffmann P, Thoren P (1986) Long-lasting cardiovascular depression induced by acupuncture-like stimulation of the sciatic nerve in unanaesthetized rats. Effects of arousal and type of hypertension. Acta Physiol Scand 127: 119–126

79 a. Hyde E (1989) Acupressure therapy for morning sickness. A controlled clinical trial. J Nurse Midwifery 34: 171–178

79 b. Hu S, Stern RM, Koch KL (1992) Electrical acustimulation relieves vection-induced motion sickness. Gastroenterology 102: 1854–1859

80. Illingsworth CM, Barker CT (1980) Measurement of electrical currents emerging during the regeneration of amputated finger tips in children. Clin Phys Physiol Meas 1: 87–91

81. Jaffe L, Barker AT et al (1982) The glabrous epidermis of cavies contains a powerful battery. Am J Physiol 242: R358–R366

81 a. Jansen G, Lundeberg T et al (1989) Increased survival of ischemic musculocutaneous flaps in rats after acupuncture. Acta Physiol Scand 135: 555–558

81 b. Jansen G, Lundeberg T et al (1989) Acupuncture and sensory neuropeptides increase cutaneous blood flow in rats. Neurosci Lett 97: 305–309

81 c. Janssens LA, Rogers PA, Schoen AM (1988) Acupuncture analgesia: a review. Vet Rec 122: 355–358

48

82. Jensen LB, Melsen B, Jensen SB (1979) Effect of acupuncture on headache measured by reduction in number of attacks and use of drugs. Scand J Dent Res 87: 373–380

83. Kaada B, Jorum E, Sagvolden T (1979) Analgesia induced by trigeminal nerve stimulation (electroacupuncture) abolished by nuclei raphe lesions in rats. Acupunct Electrother Res 4: 221–234

83 a. Kenyon JM (1985) Modern techniques of acupuncture, vol 3. Thorsons, Wellingsborough

83 b. Kho HG, Eijk RJ et al (1991) Acupuncture and transcutaneous stimulation analgesia in comparison with moderate-dose fentanyl anesthesia in major surgery. Clinical efficacy and influence on recovery and morbidity. Anesthesia 46: 129–135

84. Kim KC, Yount RA (1974) The effect of acupuncture on migraine headache. Am J Chin Med 2: 407–411

85. Kiser RS, Khatam MJ et al (1983) Acupuncture relief of chronic pain syndrome correlates with increased plasma met-enkephalin concentrations. Lancet II: 1394–1396

86. Kobori M, Mera H, Takeshige C (1986) Nature of acupuncture point and non-point stimulation produced analgesia after lesion of analgesia inhibitory system. [in Japanese (English abstract)] In: Takeshige C (ed) Studies on the mechanism of acupuncture analgesia based on animal experiments. Showa University Press, Tokyo, p 598

87. Kroenig R, Oleson TD (1984) Rapid narcotic detoxification in chronic pain patients treated with auricular electroacupuncture and naloxone. Int J Addict 20: 725–740

87 a. Kubiena G (1989) Considerations on the concept of placebo in acupuncture. Reflections on the usefulness, ethical justification, standardization and differentiated application of placebo in acupuncture. Wien Klin Wochenschr 101: 362–367

88. Lagerweij E, Van Ree J et al (1984) The twitch in horses: a variant of acupuncture. Science 225: 1172–1173

89. Laitinen J (1975) Acupuncture for migraine prophylaxis: a prospective clinical study with six months follow-up. Am J Chin Med 3: 271–274

90. Laitinen J (1976) Acupuncture and transcutaneous electric stimulation in the treatment of chronic sacrolumbalgia and ischialgia. Am J Chin Med 4: 169–175

90 a. Lazorthes Y, Esquerre JP et al (1990) Acupuncture meridians and radiotracers. Pain 40: 109–112

90 b. Le Bars D, Besson JM et al (1979) Diffuse noxious inhibitory controls (DNIC). II. Lack of effect on non-convergent neurones, supraspinal involvement and theoretical implications. Pain 6: 305–327

91. Lee DC, Clifford DH et al (1979) Can naloxone inhibit the cardiovascular effect of acupuncture? Can Anaesth Soc J 26: 410–414

91 a. Lee JH, Beitz AJ (1993) The distribution of brain-stem and spinal

nuclei associated with different frequencies of electroacupuncture analgesia. Pain 52: 11–28

91 b. Lee JH, Beitz AJ (1992) Electroacupuncture modifies the expression of c-fos in the spinal cord induced by noxious stimulation. Brain Res 577: 80–91

92. Lee Peng CH, Yang MMP et al (1978) Endorphin release: a possible mechanism of AA. Comp Med East West 6: 57–60

93. Lee PK, Andersen TW et al (1975) Treatment of chronic pain with acupuncture. J Am Med Assoc 232: 1133–1135

93 a. Lee YH, Lee WC et al (1992) Acupuncture in the treatment of renal colic. J Urol 147: 16–118

94. Lee SC, Yin SJ, Lee ML, Tsai WJ (1982) Effects of acupuncture on serum cortisol level and dopamine beta-hydroxylase activity in normal Chinese. Am J Chin Med 10: 62–69

94 a. Leong RJ, Chernow B (1988) The effects of acupuncture on operative pain and the hormonal responses to stress. Int Anesthesiol Clin 26: 213–217

95. Leung PC (1979) Treatment of low back pain with acupuncture. Am J Chin Med 7: 372–378

95 a. Lewis IH, Pryn SJ et al (1991) Effect of P 6 acupressure on postoperative vomiting in children undergoing outpatient strabismus correction. Br J Anesth 67: 73–78

96. Lewith GT, Machin D (1983) On the evaluation of the clinical effects of acupuncture. Pain 16: 111–127

97. Lewith GT, Field J, Machin D (1983) Acupuncture compared with placebo in post-herpetic pain. Pain 17: 361–368

98. Liao SJ (1978) Recent advances in the understanding of acupuncture. Yale J Biol Med 51: 55–65

99. Liao YY, Seto K, Saito H et al (1979) Effect of acupuncture on adrenocortical hormone production: variation in the ability for adrenocortical hormone production in relation to the duration of acupuncture stimulation. Am J Chin Med 7: 362–371

99 a. List T (1992) Acupuncture in the treatment of patients with craniomandibular disorders. Comparative, longitudinal and methodological studies. Swed Dent J Suppl 87: 152–159

99 b. List T, Hekimo (1992) Acupuncture and occlusal splint therapy in the treatment of craniomandibular disorders II. A one-year follow up study. Acta Odontol Scand 50: 375–385

99 c. List T, Andersson S et al (1992) Acupuncture and occlusive splint therapy in the treatment of craniomandibular disorders. I. A comparative study. Swed Dent J 16: 125–141

100. Lim TW, Loh T, Kranz H, Scott D (1977) Acupuncture effect on normal subjects. Med J Aust 26: 440–442

100 a. Liu X, Zhu B et al (1986) Relationship between electroacupuncture analgesia and descending pain inhibitory mechanism of nucleus raphe magnus. Pain 24: 383–396

101. Loh L, Nathan PW et al (1984) Acupuncture versus medical treatment for migraine and muscle tension headaches. J Neurol Neurosurg Psychiatry 47: 333–337
102. Low SA (1974) Acupuncture and heroin withdrawal. Med J Aust 2: 341
103. Loy TT (1983) Treatment of cervical spondylosis. Med J Aust 2: 32–34
104. Lu GW (1983) Characteristics of afferent fiber innervation on acupuncture point zusanli. Am J Physiol 245: R 606–R 612
105. Lung CH, Sun AC, Tsao CJ et al (1978) An observation of the humoral factor in acupuncture analgesia in rats. Am J Chin Med 2: 203–205
106. Lynn B, Perl ER (1977) Failure of acupuncture to produce localized analgesia. Pain 3: 339–351
107. Macdonald AJR, Macrae KD et al (1983) Superficial acupuncture in the relief of chronic low back pain. Ann R Coll Surg Engl 65: 44–46
108. Madden J, Akil H, Barchas JD et al (1977) Stress induced parallel changes in central opioid levels and pain responsiveness in rat. Nature 265: 358–360
109. Malizia F, Paolucci D et al (1979) Electroacupuncture and peripheral beta-endorphin and ACTH levels. Lancet II: 535–536
110. Man PL, Chuang MY (1980) Acupuncture in methadone withdrawal. Int J Addict 15: 921–926
111. Martelete M, Fiori AM (1985) Comparative study of the analgesic effect of transcutaneous nerve stimulation (TNS), electroacupuncture (EA), and meperidine in the treatment of postoperative pain. Acupunct Electrother Res 10: 183–193
112. Marx JL (1977) Analgesia: how the body inhibits pain perception. Science 196: 471
113. Masala A, Satta G, Alagna S et al (1983) Suppression of electroacupuncture (EA)-induced beta-endorphin and ACTH release by hydrocortisone in man. Absence of effects on EA-induced anaesthesia. Acta Endocrinol (Copenh) 103: 469–472
114. Matsumoto T, Levy B, Ambruso V (1974) Clinical evaluation of acupuncture. Am Surg 40: 400–405
115. Mayer DJ, Watkins LR (1984) Multiple endogenous opiate and nonopiate analgesia systems. In: Kruger L (ed) Advances in pain research and therapy, vol 6. Raven, New York, pp 253–276
116. Mayer DJ, Price DD, Raffii A (1977) Antagonism of acupuncture analgesia in man by the narcotic antagonist naloxone. Brain Res 121: 368–372
117. McCarroll GD, Rowley BA (1979) An investigation of the existence of electrically located acupuncture points. IEEE Trans Biomed Eng 26: 177–181
118. Mcdevitt L, Fortner P, Pomeranz B (1987) Application of weak electric field to the hindpaw enhances sciatic motor nerve regeneration in the adult rat. Brain Res 416: 308–314
119. McLennan H, Gilfillan K, Heap Y (1977) Some pharmacological observations on the analgesia induced by acupuncture. Pain 3: 229–238

120. Melzack R (1984) Acupuncture and related forms of folk medicine. In: Wall PD, Melzack R (eds) Textbook of pain. Churchill Livingstone, Edinburgh, pp 691–701
121. Melzack R, Katz J (1984) Auriculotherapy fails to relieve chronic pain. JAMA 251: 1041–1043
122. Melzack R, Wall PD (1965) Pain mechanism: a new theory. Science 150: 971–979
123. Melzack R, Stillwell DM, Fox EJ (1977) Trigger points and acupuncture points for pain: correlations and implications. Pain 3: 3–23
124. Mezey E, de Weid D et al (1978) Evidence for pituitary-brain transport of a behaviourally potent ACTH analogue. Life Sci 22: 831–838
125. Mizuno T (1986) The nature of acupuncture point investigation by evoked potential from the dorsal periaqueductal central grey in acupuncture afferent pathway. [in Japanese (English summary)] In: Takeshige C (ed) Studies on the mechanism of acupuncture analgesia based on animal experiments. Showa University Press, Tokyo, p 425
126. Murai M, Takeshige C et al (1986) Correlation between individual variations in effectiveness of acupuncture analgesia and that in contents of brain endogenous morphine-like factors. [in Japanese (English summary)] In: Takeshige C (ed) Studies on the mechanism of acupuncture analgesia based on animal experiments. Showa University Press, Tokyo, p 542
126 a. Naeser Ma, Alexander MP et al (1994) Acupuncture in the treatment of paralysis in chronic and acute stroke patients. Improvement correlated with specific CT scan lesion sites. Age and Ageing (in press)
126 b. Naeser MA, Alexander MP et al (1994) Acupuncture in the treatment of hand paresis in chronic and acute stroke patients. Improvement observed in all cases. Clin Rehabil (in press)
126 c. Naeser MA, Alexander MP et al (1992) Real versus sham acupuncture in the treatment of paralysis in acute stroke patients. A CT scan lesion site study. J Neurol Rehabil 6: 163–173
127. Ng LK, Donthill TC, et al (1975) Modification of morphine withdrawal syndrome in rats following transauricular electrostimulation. Biol Psychiatry 10: 575–580
128. Nakatani Y, Yamashita K (1977) Ryodoraku acupuncture. Ryodoraku Research Institute, Osaka
129. Nappi G, Faccinetti F et al (1982) Different releasing effects of traditional manual acupuncture and electroacupuncture on propiocortin-related peptides. Acupunct Electrother Res Int J 7: 93–103
130. Nogier PFM (1972) Treatise of auriculotherapy. Moulin-les-Metz, Maisonneuve, France
131. Noodergraaf, Silage D (1973) Electroacupuncture. IEEE Trans Biochem Eng 20: 364–366
132. Nuccitelli R (ed) (1986) Ionic currents in development (39 papers by various authors). Liss, New York

133. Oleson TD, Kroenig RJ, Bresler DE (1980) An experimental evaluation of auricular diagnosis: the somatotopic mapping of musculoskeletal pain at acupuncture points. Pain 8: 217–229

133 a. Omura Y (1989) Basic electrical parameters for safe and effective electro-therapeutics (electro-acupuncture, TES, TENMS, TEMS, TENS and electromagnetic field stimulation) for pain, neuromuscular skeletal problems, and circulatory disturbances. Acup Electrother Res 12: 201–225

133 b. Patel M, Gutzwiller F et al (1989) A meta-analysis of acupuncture for chronic pain. Int J Epidemiol 18: 900–906

134. Patel N, Poo MM (1982) Orientation of neurite growth by extracellular electric fields. J Neurosci 2: 483–496

135. Patterson MA (1974) Electroacupuncture in alcohol and drug addictions. Clin Med 81: 9–13

136. Peets J, Pomeranz B (1985) Acupuncture-like transcutaneous electrical nerve stimulation analgesia is influenced by spinal cord endorphins but not serotonin: an intrathecal pharmacological study. In: Fields H et al (eds) Advances in pain research and therapy. Raven, New York, pp 519–525

137. Peets J, Pomeranz B (1987) Studies of suppression of nocifensive reflexes using tail flick electromyograms and intrathecal drugs in barbiturate anaesthetized rats. Brain Res 416: 301–307

138. Peets J, Pomeranz B (1978) CXBX mice deficient in opiate receptors show poor electroacupuncture analgesia. Nature 273: 675–676

139. Pert A, Dionne R, Ng L, Pert C et al (1981) Alterations in rat central nervous system endorphins following transauricular electroacupuncture. Brain Res 224: 83–93

140. Pertovaara A, Kemppainen P et al (1982) Dental analgesia produced by non-painful, low-frequency stimulation is not influenced by stress or reversed by naloxone. Pain 13: 379–384

141. Petrie JP, Langley GB (1983) Acupuncture in the treatment of chronic cervical pain. A pilot study. Clin Exp Rheumatol 1: 33–335

141 a. Philp T, Shah PJ et al (1988) Acupuncture in the treatment of bladder instability. Br J Urol 61: 490–493

142. Pin Luo C, Takeshige C et al (1986) Inhibited region by analgesia inhibitory system in acupuncture non-point stimulation produced analgesia. [in Japanese (English summary)] In: Takeshige C (ed) Studies on the mechanism of acupuncture analgesia based on animal experiments. In: Takeshige C (ed) Showa University Press, Tokyo, p 613

143. Pomeranz B (1981) Neural mechanisms of acupuncture analgesia. In: Lipton S (ed) Persistent pain, vol 3. Academic, New York, pp 241–257

144. Pomeranz B (1985) Relation of stress-induced analgesia to acupuncture analgesia. In: Kelly J (ed) Stress-induced analgesia. Ann NY Acad Sci: 444–447

145. Pomeranz B (1986) Effects of applied DC fields on sensory nerve sprouting and motor-nerve regeneration in adult rats. In: Nuccitelli R (ed) Ionic currents in development. Liss, New York pp 251–258

146. Pomeranz B (1987) Acupuncture neurophysiology. In: Adelman G (ed) Encyclopedia of neuroscience. Birkhauser, Boston pp 6–7

147. Pomeranz B, Bibic L (1988) Naltrexone, an opiate antagonist, prevents but does not reverse the analgesia produced by electroacupuncture. Brain Res 452: 227–231

147 a. Pomeranz B, Campbell JJ (1993) Weak electric field accelerates motonenron regeneration in the sciatic nerve of ten month old rats. Brain Res 603: 271–278

148. Pomeranz B, Cheng R (1979) Suppression of noxious responses in single neurons of cat spinal cord by electroacupuncture and its reversal by the opiate antagonist naloxone. Exp Neurol 64: 327–341

149. Pomeranz B, Chiu D (1976) Naloxone blocks acupuncture analgesia and causes hyperalgesia: endorphin is implicated. Life Sci 19: 1757–1762

150. Pomeranz B, Nguyen P (1986) Intrathecal diazepam suppresses nociceptive reflexes and potentiates electroacupuncture effects in pentobarbital rats. Neurosci Lett 77: 316–320

151. Pomeranz B, Paley D (1979) Electroacupuncture hyalgesia is mediated by afferent nerve impulses: an electrophysiological study in mice. Exp Neurol 66: 398–402

151 a. Pomeranz B, Stux G (1989) Scientific bases of acupuncture. Springer, Berlin Heidelberg New York

152. Pomeranz B, Warma N (1988) Potentiation of analgesia by two repeated electroacupuncture treatments: the first opioid analgesia potentiates a second non-opioid analgesia response. Brain Res 452: 232–236

153. Pomeranz B, Cheng R, Law P (1977) Acupuncture reduces electrophysiological and behavioural responses to noxious stimuli: pituitary is implicated. Exp Neurol 54: 172–178

154. Pomeranz B, Mullen M, Markus H (1984) Effect of applied electrical fields on sprouting of intact saphenous nerve in adult rat. Brain Res 303: 331–336

155. Pontinen PJ (1979) Acupuncture in the treatment of low back pain and sciatica. Acupunct Electrother Res Int J 4: 53–57

156. Price DD, Rafii A et al (1984) A psychophysical analysis of acupuncture analgesia. Pain 19: 27–42

156 a. Rieb L, Pomeranz B (1992) Alterations in electric pain thresholds by use of acupuncture-like TENS in pain-free subjects. Phys Ther 72: 658–668

157. Reichmanis M, Marino AA, Becker RO (1975) Electrical correlates of acupuncture points. IEEE Trans Biomed Eng 22: 533–555

158. Reichmanis M, Marino AA, Becker RO (1979) Laplace plane analysis of impedence on the H meridian. Am J Chin Med 7: 188–193

159. Research Group Peking Med Coll (1974) The role of some neurotransmitters of brain in finger acupuncture analgesia. Sci Sin 17: 112–130

160. Richardson PH, Vincent CA (1986) Acupuncture for the treatment of pain: a review of evaluative research. Pain 24: 15–40

160 a. Richter A, Herbitz J, Hjalmarson A (1991) Effect of acupuncture in patients with angina pectoris. Eur Heart J 12: 178–182

161. Rossier J, Guillemin R, Bloom FE (1977) Foot shock-induced stress increases β endorphin levels in blood but not brain. Nature 270: 618–620

162. Roy BP, Cheng R, Pomeranz B et al (1980) Pain threshold and brain endorphin levels in genetically obese ob/ob and opiate receptor deficient CXBK mice. In: Way EL (ed) Exogenous and endogenous opiate agonists and antagonists. Pergamon, Elmsford, p 297

163. Sainsbury MJ (1974) Acupuncture in heroin withdrawal. Med J Aust 3: 102–105

164. Salar G, Trabucchi M et al (1981) Effect of transcutaneous electrotherapy on CSF beta endorphin content in patients without pain problems. Pain 10: 169–172

165. Sato A, Sato Y, Schmidt RF (1986) Catecholamine secretion and adrenal nerve activity in response to movements of normal and inflamed knee joints in cats. J Physiol (Lond) 375: 611–624

166. Sato T, Takeshige C (1986) Morphine analgesia caused by activation of spinal acupuncture afferent pathway in the anterolateral tract. [in Japanese (English summary)] In Takeshige C (ed) Studies on the mechanism of acupuncture analgesia based on animal experiments. Showa University Press, Tokyo p 673

167. Sato T, Usami S, Takeshige C (1986) Role of the arcuate nucleus of the hypothalamus as the descending pain-inhibitory system in acupuncture point and non-point produced analgesia. [in Japanese (English summary)] In: Takeshige C (ed) Studies on the mechanism of acupuncture analgesia based on animal experiments. Showa University Press, Tokyo, p 627

168. Sawynok J, Pinsky C, Labella FS (1979) Minireview on the specificity of naloxone as an opiate antagonist. Life Sci 25: 1621–1632

169. Schmidt RF (1971) Presynaptic inhibitions in the vertebrate central nervous system. Ergebn Physiol 63: 20–86

170. Severson L, Merkoff RA, Chun HH (1977) Heroin detoxification with acupuncture and electrical stimulation. Int J Addict 12: 911–922

171. Shen E, Ma WH, Lan C (1978) Involvement of descending inhibition in the effect of acupuncture on the splanchnically evoked potentials in the orbital cortex of cat. Sci Sin 21: 677–685

172. Shimizu S, Takeshige C et al (1986) Relationship between endogenous morphine like factor and serotonergic system in analgesia of acupuncture anesthesia. [in Japanese (English summary)] In: Takeshige C (ed) Studies on the mechanism of acupuncture analgesia based on animal experiments. Showa University Press, Tokyo, p 700

173. Shimizu T, Koja T et al (1981) Effects of methysergide and naloxone on analgesia produced by peripheral electrical stimulation in mice. Brain Res 208: 463–467

174. Shu R, Pomeranz B et al (1995) Electrical impedance measurements of human skin at acupuncture points and changes produced by needling. (to be published)

174 a. Simon J, Giraud G et al (1988) Acupuncture meridians demystified. Contributions of radiotracer methodology. Presse Med 17: 1341–1344

175. Sjolund B, Terenius L, Eriksson M (1977) Increased cerebrospinal fluid levels of endorphins after electroacupuncture. Acta Physiol Scand 100: 382–384

175 a. Smith MO, Khan I (1988) An acupuncture program for the treatment of drug-addicted persons. Bull Narc 40: 35–41

176. Sjolund BH, Erikson BE (1979) The influence of naloxone on analgesia produced by peripheral conditioning stimulation. Brain Res 173: 295–301

177. Sodipo JO, Gilly H, Pauser G (1981) Endorphins: mechanism of acupuncture analgesia. Am J Chin Med 9: 249–258

178. Spoerel W (1976) Acupuncture in chronic pain. Am J Chin Med 4: 267–279

179. Stacher G, Wancura I et al (1975) Effect of acupuncture on pain threshold and pain tolerance determined by electrical stimulation of the skin: a controlled study. Am J Chin Med 3: 143–146

179 a. Stux G, Pomeranz B (1987) Acupuncture: textbooks and atlas. Springer, Berlin Heidelberg New York

180. Sung YF, Kutner MH et al (1977) Comparison of the effects of acupuncture and codeine on postoperative dental pain. Anesth Analg 56: 473–478

181. Takahashi G, Mera H, Kobori M (1986) Inhibitory action on analgesic inhibitory system and augmenting action on naloxone reversal analgesia of D-phenylalanine. [in Japanese (English summary)] In: Takeshige C (ed) Studies on the mechanism of acupuncture analgesia based on animal experiments. Showa University Press, Tokyo, p 608

182. Takeshige C (1985) Differentiation between acupuncture and non-acupuncture points by association with an analgesia inhibitory system. Acupunct Electrother Res 10: 195–203

182 a. Takeshige C, Tsuchiya M et al (1991) Dopaminergic transmission in the arcuate nucleus to produce acupuncture analgesia in correlation with the pituitary gland. Brain Res Bull 26: 113–122

182 b. Takeshige C, Zhao WH, Guo SY (1991) Convergence from the pre-optic area and arcuate nucleus to the median eminence in acupuncture and nonacupuncture stimulation analgesia. Brain Res Bull 26: 771–778

182 c. Takeshige C, Oka K et al (1993) The acupuncture point and its connecting central pathway for producing acupuncture analgesia. Brain Res Bull 30: 53–67

182 d. Takeshige C, Nakamura A et al (1992) Positive feedback action of pituitary beta-endorphin on acupuncture analgesia afferent pathway. Brain Res Bull 29: 37–44

182 e. Takeshige C, Kobori M et al (1992) Analgesia inhibitory system involvement in nonacupuncture point stimulation produced analgesia. Brain Res Bull 28: 379–391

183. Takishima T, Mue S, Tamura G et al (1982) The bronchodilating effect of acupuncture in patients with acute asthma. Ann Allergy 48: 44–49

184. Tanaka M (1986) Studies on analgesic enhancement by D-phenylalanine. [in Japanese (English summary)] In: Takeshige C (ed) Studies on the mechanism of acupuncture analgesia based on animal experiments. Showa University Press, Tokyo, p 440

185. Tashkin D, Kroenig R et al (1977) Comparison of real and simulated acupuncture and isoproteranol in comparison to methacholine-induced asthma. Ann Allergy 39: 379–387

186. Tashkin D, Kroenig R et al (1985) A controlled trial of real and simulated acupuncture in the management of chronic asthma. J Allergy Clin Immunol 76: 855–864

186 a. Tavola T, Gala C et al (1992) Traditional Chinese acupuncture in tension-type headache: a controlled study. Pain 48: 329–332

187. Tay AA, Tseng CK, Pace NL et al (1982) Failure of narcotic antagonist to alter electroacupuncture modification of halothane anaesthesia in the dog. Can Anaesth Soc J 29: 231–235

187 a. Ter Riet G, Kleijnen J, Knipschild P (1990) A meta-analysis of studies into the effect of acupuncture on addiction. Br J Gen Pract 40: 379–382

187 b. Ter Riet G, Kleijnen J, Knipschild P (1990) Acupuncture and chronic pain: a criteria based meta-analysis. J Clin Epidemiol 43: 1191–1199

188. Toda K, Ichioka M (1978) Electroacupuncture: relations between forelimb afferent impulses and suppression of jaw opening reflex in the rat. Exp Neurol 61: 465–470

189. Thoren P, Floras JS et al (1989) Endorphins and exercise: physiological mechanisms and clinical implications. Med Sci Sports Exerc 22: 417–428

190. Travell J, Rinzler SH (1952) Myofascial genesis of pain. Postgrad Med J 11: 425–434

191. Travell J, Simmons D (1983) Myofascial pain and dysfunction. The trigger point manual. William and Wilkins, Baltimore

191 a. Tsai HY, Lin JG, Inoki R (1989) Further evidence for possible analgesic mechanism of electroacupuncture: Effects of neuropeptides and serotonergic neurons in rat spinal cord. Jpn J Pharmacol 49: 181–185

192. Tseng HL, Chang LT et al (1958) Electrical conductance and temperature of the cutaneous acupuncture points: a study of normal readings and bodily distributions. [in Chinese] J Trad Chin Med 12: 559–563

193. Tseng LF, Loh HH, Li CH (1976) Effects of systemic administration of endorphins. Nature 263: 239–240

194. Tsunoda Y, Ikezono E et al (1980) Antagonism of acupuncture analgesia by naloxone in unconscious man. Bull Tokyo Med Dent 27: 89–94

195. Usami S, Takeshige C (1986) The difference in analgesia producing central pathway of stress-induced analgesia and that of acupuncture point and non-point produced analgesia. [in Japanese (English abstract)] In: Takeshige C (ed) Studies on the mechanism of acupuncture analgesia based on animal experiments. Showa University Press, Tokyo, p 638

196. Vacca-Galloway LL et al (1985) Alterations of immunoreactive substance P and enkephalins in rat spinal cord after electroacupuncture. Peptides 6 [Suppl 1]: 177–188

196 a. Vernejoul P de, Darras JC et al (1985) Etude des meridiens d'acupuncture par les traceurs radioactifs. Bull Acad Natl Med (Paris) 169: 1071–1075

197. Vincent CA, Richardson PH (1986) The evaluation of therapeutic acupuncture: concepts and methods. Pain 24: 1–13

197 a. Vincent CA, Richardson PH et al (1989) The significance of needle placement site in acupuncture. J Psychosom Res 33: 489–496

197 b. Vincent CA (1989) A controlled trial of the treatment of migraine by acupuncture. Clin J Pain 5: 305–312

198. Walker JB, Katz RL (1981) Non-opioid pathways suppress pain in humans. Pain 11: 347–354

199. Wall PD (1972) An eye on the needle. New Sci July 20, pp 129–131

200. Wall PD (1974) Acupuncture revisited. New Sci Oct 3, pp 31–34

201. Wang K, Yao S, Xian Y, Hou Z (1985) A study on the receptive field of acupoints and the relationship between characteristics of needle sensation and groups of afferent fibres. Sci Sin 28: 963–971

201 a. Wang Q, Mao L, Han J (1990) The arcuate nucleus of hypothalamus mediates low but not high frequency electroacupuncture in rats. Brain Res 513: 60–66

201 b. Wang Q, Mao L, Han J (1990) The role of periaqueductal grey in mediation of analgesia produced by different frequencies electroacupuncture stimulation in rats. Int J Neurosci 53: 167–172

201 c. Warwick-Evan LA, Masters IJ, Redstone SB (1991) A double-blind placebo controlled evaluation of acupressure in the treatment of motion sickness. Aviat Space Environ Med 62: 776–778

201 d. Washburn A, Keenon P, Nazareno J (1990) Preliminary findings: study of acupuncture assisted heroin detoxification. Multicultural Inquiry Res on AIDS Q Newsletter 4: 3–6

202. Watkins LR, Mayer DJ (1982) Organization of endogenous opiate and non-opiate pain control systems. Science 216: 1185–1192

203. Watson SJ, Barchas JD (1979) Anatomy of the endogenous opioid peptides and related substances. In: Beers RF (ed) Mechanisms of pain and analgesic compounds. Raven, New York, pp 227–237

204. Wen HL (1977) Fast detoxification of heroin addicts and electrical stimulation in combination with naloxone. Comp Med East West 5: 257–263

205. Wen HL, Cheung SYC (1973) Treatment of drug addiction by acupuncture and electrical stimulation. Asian J Med 9: 138–141

206. Wen HL, Teo SW (1974) Experience in the treatment of drug addiction by electroacupuncture. Mod Med Asia 11: 23–24

207. Wen HL, Ho WK, Wong HK et al (1978) Reduction of adrenocorticotropic hormone (ACTH) and cortisol in drug addicts treated by acupuncture and electrical stimulation (AES). Comp Med East West 6: 61–66

208. Wen HL, Ho WK, Ling N, Ma L, Chao GH (1979) Influence of electro-acupuncture on naloxone-induced morphine withdrawal. II. Elevation of immunoassayable beta-endorphin activity in the brain but not the blood. Am J Chin Med 7: 237–240

209. Wen HL, Ho WK, Ling N et al (1980) Immunoassayable beta-endorphin level in the plasma and CSF of heroin addicted and normal subjects before and after electroacupuncture. Am J Chin Med 8: 154–159

210. Willer JC, Boureau F et al (1982) Comparative effects of EA and TENS on the human blink reflex. Pain 14: 267–278

211. Woolf CJ (1984) Transcutaneous and implanted nerve stimulation. In: Wall PD, Melzack R (eds) Textbook of pain. Churchill Livingstone, Edinburgh, pp 679–690

212. Woolf CJ, Fitzgerald M (1982) Do opioid peptides mediate a presynaptic control of C-fiber transmission in the rat spinal cord. Neurosci Lett 29: 67–72

213. Woolf CJ, Barrett G et al (1977) Naloxone reversible peripheral electroanalgesia in intact and spinal rats. Eur J Pharmacol 451: 311–314

214. Woolf CJ, Mitchell D et al (1978) Failure of naloxone to reverse peripheral TENS analgesia in patients suffering from trauma. S Afr Med J 53: 179–180

215. Woolf CJ, Mitchell J, Barrett GD (1980) Antinociceptive effect of peripheral segmental electric stimulation in the rat. Pain 8: 237–252

215 a. Wu CC, Jong SB (1989) Radionuclide venography of lower limbs by subcutaneous injection: comparison with venography by intravenous injection. Ann Nucl Med 3: 125–131

215 b. Wu CC, Jong SB et al (1990) Subcutaneous injection of 99m TC pertechnetate at acupuncture points K3 and B60. Radioisotopes 39: 261–263

216. Wu C (1984) An experience on electroacupuncture therapy of facial palsy. (abstract) Proceedings of the Second National Symposium on Acupuncture and Moxibustion. All China Society of Acupuncture, Beijing p 42

216 a. Wu DZ (1990) Acupuncture and neurophysiology. Clin Neurol Neurosurg 92: 13–25

217. Xie GX, Han JS, Hollt V (1983) Electroacupuncture analgesia blocked by microinjection of anti-beta-endorphin antiserum into periaqueductal grey of the rabbit. Int J Neurosci 18: 287–291

218. Yaksh TL, Noueihed R (1985) The physiology and pharmacology of spinal opiates. Annu Rev Pharmacol Toxicol 25: 433–462

218a. Yang ZL, Cai TW, Wu JL (1989) Acupuncture and emotion; the influence of acupuncture anesthesia on the sensory and emotional components of pain. J Gen Psychol 116: 247–258

219. Yao TS, Andersson S, Thoren P (1982) Long lasting cardiovascular depression induced by acupuncture-like stimulation of the sciatic nerve in unanaesthetized spontaneous hypertensive rat. Brain Res 240: 77–85

220. Ye W, Feng X, Shen E (1984) Evaluation of the role played by different monoaminergic descending pathways in acupuncture analgesia effects in rats. (Abstract) Proceedings of the Second National Symposium on Acupuncture and Moxibustion, All China Society of Acupuncture. Beijing, p 416

220a. Yentis SM, Bissonnetle B (1991) P 6 acupuncture and postoperative vomiting after tonsillectomy in children. Br J Anesth 67: 779–780

220b. Yentis SM, Bissonnetle B (1992) Ineffectiveness of acupuncture and droperidol in preventing vomitting following strabismus repair in children. Can J Anesth 39: 151–154

221. Yi CC, Lu TH, Wu SH, Tsou K (1977) A study on the release of tritiated 5HT from brain during acupuncture and morphine analgesia. Sci Sinica 20: 113–124

222. Yue SJ (1978) Acupuncture for chronic back and neck pain. Acupunct Electrother Res Int J 3: 323–324

223. Yuen RWM, Vaughan RJ et al (1976) The response to acupuncture therapy in patients with chronic disabling pain. Med J Aust 1: 862–865

223a. Zheng M, Yang SG, Zou B (1988) Electroacupuncture markedly increases proenkephalin mRNA in rat striatun & pituitary. Sci Sin B 31: 81–86

223b. Zao FY, Han JS et al (1987) Acupuncture analgesia in impacted last molar extraction. Effect of clomipramine and pargyline. In: Han JS (ed) The neurochemical basis of pain relief by acupuncture. A collection of papers 1973–1989. Beijing Medical Science, Beijing, pp 96–97

223c. Zhang WH, Shen YC (1981) Change in levels of monoamine neurotransmitters and their main metabolites in rat brain after electroacupuncture treatment. Int J Neurosci 15: 147–149

223d. Zhang AZ (1980) Endorphin and analgesia research in the People's Republic of China (1975–1979). Acupunct Electrother Res Int J 5: 131–146

224. Zhou ZF, Du MY, Han JS et al (1981) Effect of intracerebral microinjection of naloxone on acupuncture- and morphine-analgesia in the rabbit. Sci Sin 24: 1166–1178

225. Zou K, Yi QC, Wu SX, Lu YX et al (1980) Enkephalin involvement in acupuncture analgesia. Sci Sin 23: 1197–1207

225a. Zou K (1987) Neurochemical mechanisms of acupuncture analgesia. Pain Headache 9: 266-282

3 Background and Theory of Traditional Chinese Medicine

G. STUX

3.1 Tao, Yin and Yang

Around 200 years B.C. the basic tenets of Chinese medicine were recorded in a classic work, the **Huang Di Nei Jing,** the Yellow Emperor's textbook of physical medicine. The Chinese doctors of ancient times had a traditional theory that was based on a philosophical view of nature. They saw man as an integral part of nature and in a state of intensive interaction with his environment. Nature is in a constant state of change and continuous development.

The Chinese did not regard these developments as the work of a divine creator but as the expression of inherent conformity with a natural law, which they called **Tao** (pronounced Dao).

The essential nature of Tao was described in the 5th century B.C. by Laotse in the **Tao Te King**. The Tao is a force that creates all things. The Tao brings out the polarity between **Yin** (pronounced "inn") and **Yang** from an unstructured primal state. All things in nature develop within this field of tension between Yin and Yang. Tao remains as the continuous, creative force, the basis of all dynamic creation and transformation.

The original meaning of Yang is reflected in old the Chinese ideogram; it is the sunny (fertile) side of the hill, while Yin symbolizes the shady side.

The opposites complement each other in a dynamic process. Yin cannot exist without Yang; the two forces always combine to make up the whole. This polar system of Yin and Yang has an important role in medicine, in the description of life processes in the human body and of their pathologic disturbances (Table 3.1).

Table 3.1. System of Yin and Yang counterparts

Yin	Yang
Receptive	Creative
Earth	Heaven
Negative	Positive
Body	
Ventral	Dorsal
Internal	External
Lower	Upper
Inside	Surface
Internal organs	Skin
Functions	
Hypofunction	Hyperfunction
Deficiency **Energy**	Excess
Inadequate blood flow	Hyperemia
Cold	Heat
Degeneration	Infection

Chinese ideas of physiology and pathology are based on precise empirical observations linked up by systems of theories.

3.2 The Vital Energy, Life Force: Qi

Tao as the creative force gives rise in the dynamic polarity between Yin and Yang to the flow of life force called **"Qi."** Qi, the vital energy or life force, is omnipresent in nature and is apparent in all life in the form of change and movement. Every life process, every organic function is an expression of the action and movement of the vital energy Qi. In the body Qi accumulates in the organs and flows in channels or meridians that are called *Jing* and *Luo* in Chinese. The concept of the life force or vital energy is fundamental for the description of nature in Chinese medicine.

There are various forms of Qi with *various levels of density* in the human body:

– In the lungs Qi is received from the respiratory air. This lung Qi is called **"Zong Qi,"** "Chest Qi," "Big Qi," or "Yang Qi" because it is dynamic in its moving nature. This form of Qi is also called "gathering Qi;" it is formed in the interaction with "nutrient Qi."

- The digestive process transforms food into **"nutrient Qi"** or "Yin Qi," known in Chinese as *Ying Qi.*
- The third source of Qi in the body is the **"sourse Qi"** *"hereditary Qi,"* called in Chinese *Yuan Qi,* the vital energy each person inherits from his or her parents and which brings about the person's growth and development.

These three forms of Qi combine in the body. *Jing Qi* is the vital energy that flows through the channels *(Jing).* The functions of the organs are brought about by the Qi inherent in each. Respiration, as a function of the lungs, and digestion of food as a function of the stomach and intestine, are expressions of the Qi of each of these organs. The functions of Chinese organ systems will be described in the next chapter.

If the Qi of an organ is weakened, the function of this organ will be incomplete or faulty, but if Qi is present in excess, the result is excessive function. This is the basic theory of Chinese pathophysiology and pathogenesis.

The main functions of Qi are:

- It is the *source of movements;* not only of voluntary movements, however, but also of the movement processes involved in respiration, circulatory function, and intestinal motility.
- The *generation of warmth* in the body is a further function of Qi.
- *Psychic activity* and vitality are an expression of Qi and are known as *"Shen."*
- Further functions of Qi are the *organ functions* like the conversion of food into blood and other body fluids.
- In addition Qi also has the function of *protecting the body* from external noxious influences, e.g., climatic factors that might lead to illness. This protective function is particularly important in the prevention of illnesses. This **"protective Qi"** is known as *Wei Qi* and is concentrated mainly at the body surface.

Jing, the *life essence,* also has an important role in the description of the life processes. The life essence is regarded as the material basis of Qi. Jing is also designated as the "seed of life" and the "elementary reproductive force." The evolutive processes in the body, differentiation of the organs and growth, are also traditionally considered to reflect the action of Jing. The primary or congenital Jing arises from the union of the parental life essences, and it is this that determines the growth and development of each individual and the nature of his or her particular constitution.

Shen is another important concept in traditional Chinese medicine. It is the force of consciousness and is often translated as *"spirit."* Shen gives birth to our thoughts. It is traditionally believed to be stored in the heart and revealed in the eyes. When Shen is disturbed, the eyes become clouded, colorless and dull; the patient becomes forgetful and retarded, and the sleep pattern is upset. If the disturbance of Shen is very marked, there are also changes in the conscious state.

3.3 Pathogenesis of Chinese Medicine

According to Chinese tradition most illnesses are rooted in a disturbance of the flow of Qi; there is either an *excess* or a *deficiency* of the vital energy in the organ systems and the channels. A *stagnation* of Qi in the channels is another possible cause of illness.

Deficiency conditions (Table 3.2) are characterized by a weakness of Qi and therefore by *inadequate functioning* of the corresponding organs. The Chinese called deficiency-type disharmonies "*Xu* conditions." If there is a general weakness of the vital energy throughout the entire body, many different cardinal symptoms occur, such as pallor, cold hands and feet, immoderate coldness, low blood pressure, lack of drive, lowered activity, lack of energy. Typical illnesses that arise with disturbances involving deficiency are degenerative illnesses, diseases of old age, and mental depression.

An **excess of vital energy** leads to *excessive function* of the organ systems concerned. They are referred to as *Shi* or Yang conditions. Important symptoms in conditions of excess are plethora, flushing, acute shooting or cramp-type pain, inner uneasiness, nervousness, and overexcitement.

64

Table 3.2. Disturbances involving deficiency and excess

Deficiency of Qi; *Xu*	Excess of Qi; *Shi*
Yin condition	Yang condition
Symptoms of coldness	Symptoms of heat
Pallor	Flushing
Inadequate blood flow	Plethora
Feeling cold	Feeling hot
Slack muscles	Tense muscles
Hypofunction	Hyperfunction
Depressive illnesses	Agitation
Hypoactivity	Hyperactivity
Dull pains	Acute pains
Degenerative illnesses	Inflammatory illnesses

When the **vital energy is stagnated or blocked** the flow of Qi is disturbed, primarily in the peripheral and superficial areas of the body. The *main symptom* of a stagnation or blockage is **pain.** The usual result of this stagnation of vital energy is called *Qi Zhi Zheng* and is a state of excess. Inappropriately high muscle tone, muscle pains, myogelosis, and restricted movement are typical features of such conditions. A stagnation is often present in headache, together with an excess of Qi, leading to feelings of tension and acute pain.

Traditionally, illnesses are divided according to whether they have "internal" or "external" causes:

– Illnesses are **externally caused** when the "energy" of nature round about, e. g., in the form of *climatic influences,* acts on the weakened body, thus leading to disturbances of Qi in the channels and organs. External climatic factors are heat, cold, dryness, damp, wind, or a combination of such factors, e. g., a cold dry wind. The external causes of illnesses are traditionally believed to affect the peripheral regions and the superficial layers of the body first, particularly when the normal protective function of Qi is inadequate. **Internal causes** of disturbances of the vital energy, such as *faulty nutrition* or *mental and emotional stress,* can also lead to illness. Excessive emotions, such as fear, rage, anger, brooding, agitation and sadness, lead to a disturbance of the energy in individual organs. Disturbances of internal organs owing to deficiency or excess occur particularly when feelings arise suddenly and are especially intense and inadequately processed.

In addition to this main causes of illnesses infections, overexcitation i.e. overwork or excessive sexual activities, akumulation of plegm and trauma are described by chinese medicine.

3.4 The System of Five Phases

In addition to the system of Yin and Yang, which made it possible to understand polar processes, the system of the **"five phases,"** or "five elements," in Chinese *Wu Xing,* was introduced in the 3rd century B.C. to allow the categorization of processes with a phasic course. This system was an essential standardization of the ancient natural philosophers' view of the world. The traditional system of Chinese medicine classed widely varying natural processes and evolutionary events in this system. The five phases are wood, fire, earth, metal, and water. These basic phases are intimately interlinked, in such a way that they stimulate but also inhibit or control; each is controlled by another, while itself simultaneously controlling a third phase.

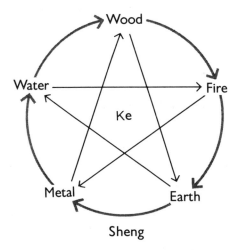

Table 3.3. The five-phase system of equivalents

Elements	Directions	Seasons	Climatic factors	Colors	Stages of development
Wood	East	Spring	Wind	Green	Birth
Fire	South	Summer	Heat	Red	Growth
Earth	Center	Latesummer	Damp	Yellow	Change
Metal	West	Autumn	Dryness	White	Harvest
Water	North	Winter	Cold	Black	Composure

Table 3.4. Classification by the five phases

Elements	Internal organs	Hollow organs	Sensory organs	Body layer	Emotion	Taste
Wood	Liver	Gallbladder	Eye	Muscle	Anger	Sour
Fire	Heart	Small intestine	Tongue	Blood vessels	Joy	Bitter
Earth	Spleen	Stomach	Mouth	Connective tissue "flesh"	Anxiety	Sweet
Metal	Lung	Large intestine	Nose	Skin	Sadness	Spicy
Water	Kidney	Urinary bladder	Ear	Bone, joints	Fear	Salty

The concept of these five phases forms a sort of abstract symbol that allows the classification of empirical observations in different fields (Table 3.3).

In medicine, the functions of internal organs, tissues, and sensory organs are classified in this way according to the five phases (Table 3.4).

3.5 Diagnosis in Traditional Chinese Medicine

The diagnostic system of Chinese medicine developed on the basis of the philosophical system of the Yin-Yang polarity and the theory of the five phases. This traditional system classes the individual signs and symptoms of illness according to diametrically opposed diagnostic criteria. Eight diagnostic criteria are known, four couples made up of polar extremes, called *Ba gang* in Chinese:

Yin and Yang
Interior and exterior   (*Li* and *Biao* in Chinese)
Deficiency and excess   (*Xu* and *Shi* in Chinese)
Cold and heat   (*Han* and *Re* in Chinese)

The symptoms of a functional disturbance or an illness are analyzed with reference to these eight diagnostic criteria. Disharmonies of the vital energy in the channels or organs and the effects of such disturbances are all described with reference to these eight polar criteria. The Chinese doctor assesses the individual symptoms and signs in categories referring to disturbances of Yin and Yang in the organs or channels, thus ascertaining "patterns of disharmony" which are called "syndromes."

The four couples of opposites used in the Chinese system of diagnosis are explained below.

Interior and Exterior

Internal disturbances, called *Li* in Chinese, are disharmonious states of the five *Zang* organs and the six *Fu* organs. The disturbances of these internal organs are frequently chronic in nature, being characterized by pains in the area of the thorax or abdomen, raised body temperature, and disturbances of the gastrointestinal function, such as retching, diarrhea, and nausea. Internal illnesses are often caused by an excess of such feelings as anxiety, fear, sadness, or excitement, or by inadequate or contaminated food.

External illnesses, called *Biao* in Chinese, are characterized by disturbances of the channels and collaterals, especially in the peripheral regions and at the surface of the body. The external disturbance is usually characterized by acute pain in the extremities, the joints, or the head, and by sensitivity to climatic factors. Typical external disturbances are peripheral neuralgia or localized joint disease. Chinese medicine considers that these are caused by external pathogenic climatic influences, such as cold, heat, damp, wind, or dryness.

Deficiency and Excess

Deficiency disturbances, or *Xu* conditions in Chinese, are characterized by a deficiency of Qi, of blood, or of Jing, the elementary essence. Deficiency-induced disturbances lead to hypofunction of organ systems. Typical symptoms of such disturbances are excessive tiredness, exhaustion, dizziness, motor retardation, pallor of the skin, tongue and mucous membranes, low blood pressure, inadequate blood perfusion, sudden profuse sweating, oliguria, and deficiency of body fluids (Table 3.5). A pale tongue and a weak pulse are important signs for the diagnosis.

The deficiency diseases are usually chronic. The most usual cause is exhaustion of Qi following the action of internal pathogenic influences over a long period.

Disturbances caused by excess, or *Shi* in Chinese, are characterized by an excessive amount of Qi or blood in organs and channels. Typical symptoms are acute pain, cramps, hypertension, plethora, increased muscle tone, and increased secretion of body fluids (Table 3.5). The most important signs are redness of the face and a strong pulse. In the psychological sector agitation, nervousness, overexcitement, restlessness, aimless activity and sleeplessness.

Table 3.5. Typical symptoms of excess and deficiency

Excess, *Shi*	Deficiency, *Xu*
Powerful muscular movements	Feeble, slow muscular movements
Agitation, hyperactivity	Tiredness, exhaustion
Loud voice	Faint voice
Upright posture	Stooping posture
Quick, vigorous way of walking	Slow gait
Hypertension	Hypotension
Hyperemia	Deficient blood perfusion
Psychologically active attitude	Psychological passivity
Excitement, mania	Depression, subdued mood
Excessive activity	Deficient activity
Short sleep period, difficulty in falling asleep	Long sleep period with disturbed sleep
Coated tongue	Little coating of tongue
Strong pulse	Weak pulse

Cold and Heat

Cold disturbances, or *Han* in Chinese, occur when external pathogenic cold takes effect in a body in which Qi is weakened. In these circumstances typical cold-type symptoms manifest themselves, such as immoderate feelings of cold, cold extremities, and pallor (Table 3.6). Cold disturbances are usually chronic. The active Yang Qi in the body becomes continuously weaker.

Heat disturbances, or *Re* in Chinese, are caused basically by increased Yang activity of the Qi in the body. Qi is responsible for the generation of heat in the body. The hyperactivity of Yang leads to exhaustion of the Yin forces and of the Yin fluids if it persists, and as a result the Yang system develops heat. Typical heat-type symptoms are high body temperature, redness, hyperemia, pain, and agitation (Table 3.6). Obstinate constipation, dark urine, a red tongue, and a fast pulse can also occur.

Table 3.6. Typical heat- and cold-type symptoms

Heat, *Re*	Cold, *Han*
Red face	Pale face
Redness of skin and mucous membranes	Pale mucous membranes
Warmness/burning of the extremities	Cold extremities
Fever	Hypothermia
Feeling hot	Feeling cold
Exacerbation of the symptoms	Exacerbation of the symptoms
by heat (e.g., in bath)	by cold
Thirst for cold drinks	Need for warm drinks
Dark, scanty urine	Dilute urine
Obstinate constipation	Watery stool
Fast pulse	Slow pulse
Red tongue	Pale tongue

Yin and Yang

Yin and Yang are the categories within Chinese thought that have universal validity and are applicable to all phenomena. Thus, the diagnostic criteria discussed above, interior – exterior, excess – deficiency, heat – cold, should be regarded as shadings of the generally valid criteria of Yin and Yang. Exterior, excess, and heat are Yang criteria, while interior, deficiency, and cold are Yin criteria.

The eight diagnostic criteria seldom occur in isolation as described, but rather in various combinations. Thus, excess and heat, two Yang criteria, often occur together. The classic phrase for a phenomenon of this kind is Yang in Yang. Excess and cold can also occur simultaneously, or deficiency and heat. Often it is necessary to apply the eight diagnostic categories to the symptoms of illness and functional disturbances of a specific Zang and Fu organs.

4 Channels, Organs, and Points

G. STUX

4.1 System of Channels and Organs

According to traditional ideas the vital energy flows through a system of channels also called meridians and regulates the body functions. It is possible to exert a direct therapeutic effect on the channels and organs, and thus in turn on body functions, by needling acupuncture points.

The **11 organs** described by Chinese medicine interact intimately with the channels. The structure and topography of the organs was subordinate in Chinese medicine. "Organs" in the Chinese sense has much more the meaning of the functions of organ systems. The functional system of the lung, for example, involves all respiratory processes, including olfactory. This is why the term **"functional systems"** is also used.

The 11 organs or functional systems were divided into 6 Yang organs and 5 Yin organs. The **6 Yang organs** are called **Fu organs** in Chinese: they are the hollow organs, i.e., large intestine, small intestine, stomach, urinary bladder, gallbladder and "Sanjiao." The functions of the Fu organs are similar to those in Western medicine. The **5 Yin organs** are the **Zang organs:** lung, heart, spleen, kidney and liver. Pericardium is not considered as a Zang organ, but it has a channel. The traditional functions of the five Zang organs are described here:

Heart *Xin* governs all other organs and regulates the flow of blood and Qi. It stores and rules the mental energy, the mind, and consciousness (Shen). According to traditional Chinese diagnosis "the heart opens to the tongue." The climatic factor is heat, and the emotion is joy or agitation.

Lung *Fei* controls the respiration and is responsible for the intake of Qi. "The clear lung Qi flows downward." The lung governs the surface of the body, the skin, and the bodyhair, and has its expression in the voice. According to traditional theory "it opens to the nose." The lung is very sensitive and vulnerable to external climatic influences.

Spleen *Pi* controls the digestion of food and is responsible for the intake of fluids. It assimilates the Qi from nutrition, transforms it and nourishes the internal organs and moves and nourishes the blood. The spleen governs the connective tissue and holds the organs in place. It opens to the mouth and is manifested in the lips.

Liver *Gan* is responsible for the movement of all body fluids. It moves the Qi and stores the blood. The liver Qi controls the movements of the body and nourishes muscles and tendons. It produces the bile, the Yang aspect. The liver nourishes the eyes. The pathogenic climatic influence is the wind. Liver needs moisture and kidney Yin. Liver disharmonies are characterized by stagnation, and often by excess.

Kidney *Shen* is the root of life (reproduction); it stores the Jing, the essence, and is the base of growth and development. It rules water (Yin aspect) and excretes the impure. Mental activity and sexual potency, *Ming Men Huo, fire of the gate of life* form the Yang aspect. The kidney nourishes the bones, joints and teeth, rules the ears and manifests in head hair. The kidney energy weakens in old age.

One Yin and one Yang organ form a **functional unit,** which involves a particular tissue, and the corresponding channels. The channel (Jing) can be compared with a branch deriving from the tree represented by the organ. The acupuncture points are situated along the channel like buds. By way of these points a therapeutic influence can be exerted on the organ function by the application of needles, heat, or massage.

A **pair of channels** consists of a Yin and a Yang channel (e.g., lung and large intestine channels) which run parallel to one another in the limbs. They are also called coupled channels, because in the peripheral areas they are coupled with connecting vessels, the **Luo connections.** Yang channels run laterally or on the dorsal side of the body, while Yin channels run medially or on the ventral side.

The 12 channels belonging to the 11 organs are termed **main channels** or "master meridians." Together with the Luo connections, which connect each Yin-Yang pair of channels, they are referred to collectively by the Chinese as the **Jing-Luo system.**

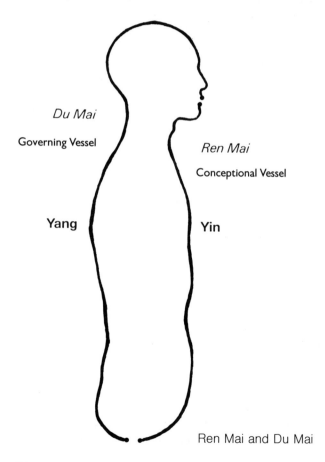

Du Mai

Governing Vessel

Ren Mai

Conceptional Vessel

Yang

Yin

Ren Mai and Du Mai

In addition to the 12 coupled main channels there are other channel systems. Among the **eight** channels that make up the system of **extraordinary channels** (*Qi Jingbamai* in Chinese), also called "irregular or marvellous channels," there are two, those with their courses on the ventral and dorsal midlines of the body, that are particularly important. The one at the front of the body, **Ren Mai,** is also referred to as the conceptional vessel. The one in the midline of the back, **Du Mai,** is the governing vessel, which counts as a Yang channel. These 2 extraordinary channels and the 12 coupled main channels together make up the **system of 14 channels** on which the 361 classic acupuncture points are situated.

The 12 main channels make up a system of three courses or cycles of channels at the body surface. One **course of channels** is made up of four main channels, two Yin and two Yang channels. One Yin-Yang pair runs in parallel course along the arm, and one along the leg. An internal branch of the channel derives from the main channel running to the corresponding Yin or Yang organ. Thus, a coupled Yin-Yang channel and the corresponding Zang and Fu organs together make up a functional and morphological unit. The Zang and Fu organs thus belong together as a functional system, while the corresponding Yin-Yang channels running in parallel are linked in the peripheral regions by way of the Luo connections.

The topography of the **three channel courses** and their connections are described below. The first course is located on the ventral side of the body, the second, on the dorsal side and the third, on the lateral side.

The **first course** is made up of the lung, large intestine, stomach, and spleen channels (see next figure). The lung channel starts at the chest wall and runs along the arm to the corner of the thumbnail. Its course is on the volar side of the arm, i.e., the inside, and it is considered to belong to the Yin polarity. The large intestine channel starts from the index finger and runs on the dorsal, or outer, side of the arm to the face; this channel is classed as part of the Yang polarity. The face is the starting point of the stomach channel, which runs ventrally down the body to the second toe. It corresponds to the Yang polarity. The spleen channel, finally, runs from the foot back to the chest wall, thus completing the first course of the channels. The course of the spleen channel is along the inside

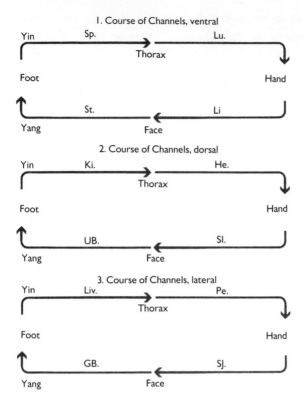

1. Course of Channels, ventral

Yin — Sp. — Thorax — Lu.
Foot — Hand
St. — Li
Yang — Face

2. Course of Channels, dorsal

Yin — Ki. — Thorax — He.
Foot — Hand
UB. — SI.
Yang — Face

3. Course of Channels, lateral

Yin — Liv. — Thorax — Pe.
Foot — Hand
GB. — SJ.
Yang — Face

of the leg and corresponds to the Yin polarity. A simple rule emerges from all this: Yin channels run on inner surfaces, i.e., ventral or medial ones, while Yang channels run along outer, i.e., dorsal or lateral surfaces.

The arrangement of the second and third courses of channels is similar to that of the first. The **second course** is sited on the dorsal side of the body and is made up of the heart, small intestine, urinary bladder, and kidney channels. The third course is made up of the channels relating to the pericardium, Sanjiao, gallbladder, and liver and is situated laterally on the body. The third course passes laterally around the middle of the body and the extremities, between the first course on the ventral side and the second course on the dorsal side.

Table 4.1. Three courses of channels

	Yin	Yang	Yang	Yin
1st course	Lung	Large intestine	Stomach	Spleen
2nd course	Heart	Small intestine	Urinary bladder	Kidney
3rd course	Pericardium	Sanjiao	Gallbladder	Liver

The three Yin channels for the lung (radial), heart (ulnar), and pericardium start from the lateral chest wall and run distally along the inside of the arm, ending at the corners of the fingernails. The three Yang channels for the large intestine (radial), small intestine (ulnar), and Sanjiao start from the hand and run along the outside of the arm to the face. The three Yang channels for the stomach (ventral), urinary bladder (dorsal), and gallbladder (lateral) start from the face and pass to the foot. The course of the channels is completed with the three Yin channels of the leg: those for spleen, kidney, and liver (Table 4.1).

Two adjacent Yang channels or two adjacent Yin channels in the same course of channels combine to make up a Yin or Yang **channel axis,** in Chinese **Chiao.** The Yang channel axes pass from the arm to the leg by way of the head and trunk, that is to say, basically downwards. The Yin channel axes have an upward direction, from the feet to the arms by way of the trunk. The Yang channel axis made up of the large intestine and the stomach channels is called the *Yang-Ming* (Table 4.2).

Table 4.2. Channel axes

Tai-Yin	Major Yin	Spleen and lung channels
Shao-Yin	Minor Yin	Kidney and heart channels
Jue-Yin	Absolute Yin	Liver and pericardium channels
Yang-Ming	Brilliant Yang	Large intestine and stomach channels
Tai-Yang	Major Yang	Small intestine and urinary bladder channels
Shao-Yang	Minor Yang	Sanjiao and gallbladder channels

The channel axes are important for diagnosis as well as for treatment. Thus, pain localized along the path of a particular channel is often treated by stimulation of points on the channel axis; in painful shoulder with pain in the area of the large intestine channel, for example, acupuncture needles are often applied at point St. 38 Tiaokou on the Yang-Ming channel axis.

4.2 Point Categories

A large number of acupuncture points can be allocated to point categories. Points with particular functions are grouped in these categories. Thirteen categories of points are known in traditional Chinese medicine. The separate point categories are presented below with reference to their semantic origin, functional significance, localization, and the links between the separate categories.

4.2.1 Shu Points or Transport Points

The Chinese word *Shu* means to convey or transport. A distinction is made between two groups of Shu points:

The 12 Shu points on the urinary bladder channel are also referred to as *Beishuxue* or **Back Shu points** (see Table 4.4). They are traditionally believed to convey the vital energy Qi to the corresponding organs. One Shu point on the urinary bladder channel is allocated to each of the organs. These points are situated 1.5 cun lateral to the center of the vertebral column in each segment. They become sensitive to pressure when the organs corresponding to them are diseased. Treatment of these Beishu points is indicated in illnesses of the organs.

In addition to the 12 Back Shu points on the urinary bladder channel, there are the 5 Shu points on each channel; these points are discussed below (Sect. 4.2.5).

4.2.2 Mu or Alarm Points

Mu means collect. The Mu, or alarm, points are situated ventrally on the trunk and are also known as **Mu front points.** One Mu front point is attributed to each internal organ. These points have a similar function to the Back Shu points, that is to say, the treatment of organ disorders, and are often used together with the Shu points. When the organs corresponding to these points are diseased, they also become sensitive to pressure, so that they are important in diagnosis, as alarm points, as well as in treatment.

4.2.3 Influential Points, Hui Xue

Apart from their other effects, the eight influential points have a specific influence on the tissues and/or organs corresponding to them. *Hui* means to assemble or collect. They are traditionally believed to be the points at which Qi for the corresponding organs or tissues is concentrated.

4.2.4 Xi-Cleft Points

Xi means cleft or space. It is traditionally believed that each Xi-cleft point is the place where the Qi is accumulated in the channel. Treatment of the Xi-cleft points (Wade-Giles: *Tsri*) is indicated in the case of acute illness of the corresponding organs or channels.

4.2.5 Five Shu Points

The five Shu points are situated in the peripheral part of each channel, distal to the elbow or knee. The peripheral position of each channel is traditionally believed to be subject to external climatic influences such as cold, heat, dryness, damp, and wind. Each of the five Shu points corresponds to one of the five phases. The positions of the five phases are different on the Yin and the Yang channels. Thus, on the Yang channels the Jing points correspond to the element metal, while on the Yin channels they correspond to wood. In addition, one Shu point on each channel corresponds to the same element as the channel as a whole. This point is called the hourly point. According to the traditional mother-and-son law there is a tonification point and a sedative point for each channel.

4.2.6 Tonification Point

The tonification point of the channel is the point preceding the hourly point, the "mother point." In the case of the lung channel the metal point is the hourly point and is preceded by the element earth (Yuan point), which is the tonification point. The Yuan point of the lung channel is Lu. 9 Taiyuan (Table 4.3).

4.2.7 Sedative Point

In contrast to the tonification point, the sedative point is the point following the hourly point; it is the "son point." In the case of the lung channel (Table 4.3) the sedative point corresponds to the element water and is the He point, Lu. 5 Chize.

4.2.8 Jing Well Point

The Jing well point (Wade-Giles: *Ting*) is the most distally situated point on any channel. *Jing* means well. The Jing point is the source of the "river" that carries the Qi.

4.2.9 Ying Point

The Ying point (Wade-Giles: *Yong* or *Jong*) is the second of the five Shu points. The translation of *Ying* is "old lake." The word now has the meaning of a slow-flowing river, because at this point the Qi coming from the well flows along slowly and is distributed

Table 4.3. Tonification and sedative points on the lung channel

Jing	Ying	Yuan	Jing	He
Lu. 11	Lu. 10	Lu. 9	Lu. 8	Lu. 5
Wood	Fire	Earth	Metal is related	Water
		Tonification point	to the lung	**Sedative point**

over a wider area. Cold is stimulated in the case of the Yang channels and heat in the case of the Yin channels (see allocation of the five points to the phases and climatic factors).

4.2.10 Yuan Source Point

The Yuan (Wade-Giles: *Yunn*) point is also called the source point and is situated in the area of the wrist or the ankle. *Yuan* means origin, source, beginning. The Yuan point is the marshalling point, the source of Qi from the coupled channel. Puncture of the Yuan source point attracts the energy of the coupled channel, because the Luo vessel coming from the Luo point of the coupled channel ends at this point.

The Yang channels have a further point, the **Shu point** (Wade-Giles: *Yu*), which corresponds to wood. *Shu* means to transport. The Qi begins to flow more rapidly at this point. On the Yin channels, the Yuan and Shu points are the same.

4.2.11 Jing Point

The Jing point (Wade-Giles: *King*) is the fourth of the five Shu points, Shu IV, and is situated proximal to the wrist or ankle. *Jing* means to pass through and signifies that the stream of Qi becomes a river at this point.

4.2.12 He Sea Point

The He points (Wade-Giles: *Ho*) are the most proximally situated of the five Shu points and are found in the areas of the elbow and knee. *He* means oneness, and this term thus implies that at this point the river of Qi flows into the sea of the body. This is where the superficial, distal course of the channel ends, giving way to the deep, proximal course. Thus, the He point provides the connection between the peripheral and the proximal parts of the channel. The He points are of decisive importance in the treatment of diseases of the internal organs. Many of the most frequently used acupuncture points are He points, for example St. 36 Zusanli, LI. 11 Quchi, and GB. 34 Yanglingquan.

4.2.13 Luo Connecting Point

The Luo or connecting point (Wade-Giles: *Lo*) is situated proximal to the Yuan point. It is the starting point for the Luo connecting vessel. The Luo point is not counted as one of the five Shu points but is a point category in its own right.

4.2.14 Confluent Points

The confluent points are on the main channels in the area of the wrist or ankle and form a link between the main channels and the extraordinary channels. These key points are traditionally believed to bring the extraordinary channels into play. Most of the key points are Luo or Yuan points.

4.3 Methods of Point Location

Accurate location of the acupuncture points is very important for the success of the treatment. Several methods of locating acupuncture points are used. Every acupuncture point is located with its own specific method. Some points can be located with the aid of more than one method. Palpation of the area concerned is important, because acupuncture points mostly become increasingly sensitive to palpation. Especially in the area of painful disorders of the locomotor system, but also in neurological disorders, points that are tender to pressure are found. These points are also needled even through they do not correspond to classic acupuncture points in their location. Such **tender points** are called **Ah Shi points** in Chinese and are indicated as local points in addition to the specific distal points. After needling acupuncture points, it is useful to check the correct position of the needle, and in the event of excessive divergence, to needle once more.

Anatomical Landmarks

Acupuncture points are located with the help of anatomical landmarks of the body, such as eyebrow, hairline, transverse crease of a joint, spinous processes of the vertebrae, mamillae, navel, and upper border of the symphysis.

Examples:
Du 13 Taodao is located between the spinous processes of the 1st and 2nd thoracic vertebrae.
Ex.1 Yintang is located between the eyebrows.

Proportional Cun Measurement

The Chinese use the cun or **"body inch"** to measure the distances on the body. The **cun** is a relative body measure. It is the distance between the transverse creases of the interphalangeal bone of the middle finger when the patient's finger is slightly flexed. The breadth of the distal phalanx of the thumb is also equal to 1 cun.

The hand has a breadth of 3 cun at the level of the proximal finger joints (4 finger breadths = 3 cun). The breadth of the index and middle fingers together is equal to 1.5 cun. The distance of the acupuncture points from transverse creases or joint clefts is measured in cun.

If the proportions of the physician and the patient are identical measurement in the physician's cun is permissible. When there is a discrepancy, for example in the treatment of children, it is difficult to size up the proportions. In Sri Lanka a device, the **cunometer,** has been developed to measure exactly in cun. It is a scissors-type instrument with four pairs of arms, their lengths in a fixed relative proportion of $1:2:3:4$. In dependence on the pair of arms used to measure off the cun, lengths of 0.25–4 cun can be set

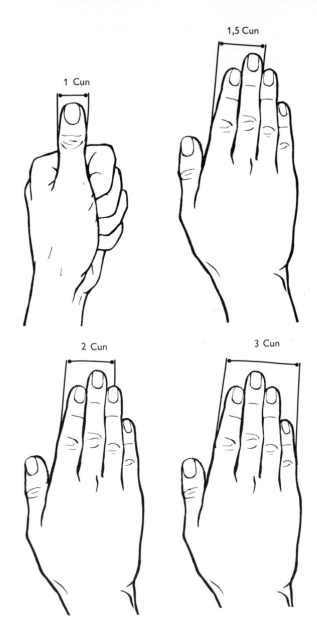

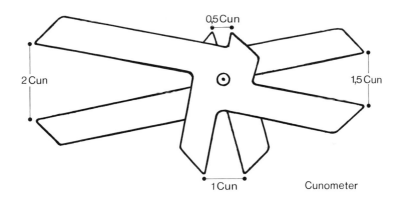

2 Cun

1,5 Cun

1 Cun   Cunometer

and used for measurement. A cunometer makes exact measurement of the individual cun possible, which is especially helpful in the treatment of children and for the beginner.

Proportional Measurement

The lengths of the various parts of the body are generally in fixed proportions to each other that can be expressed in cun (see diagram).

From the anterior to the posterior hairline, on the midline	12 cun
Between the eyebrow line and the anterior hairline	3 cun
Dorsal hairline to the prominence	3 cun
Between the two mamillae	8 cun
Between two ribs	1 cun
Between the umbilicus and the tip of the xiphoid	8 cun
Between the navel and the upper border of the symphysis	5 cun
Between the axillary fold and the transverse crease of the elbow	9 cun
Between the transverse creases of elbow and wrist	12 cun
Between the greater trochanter of the femur and the middle of the patella	19 cun
Between the middle of the patella and the tip of the lateral malleolus	16 cun

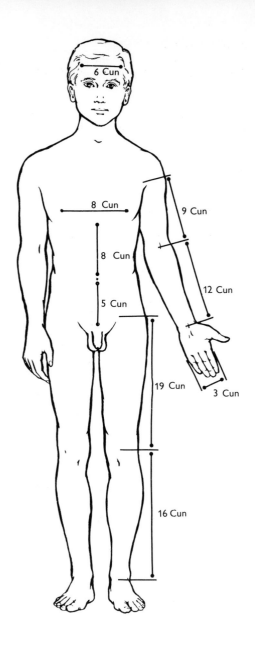

Location by Means of Specific Posture

The patient is asked to adopt a specific posture that is helpful for point location.

Examples:
LI.4 Hegu is found when the thumb is adducted, at the highest point of the resultant muscular ridge.
LI.11 Quchi is located at the lateral end of the transverse crease when the elbow is flexed to a right angle.

Location by Measurement of Skin Resistance

Many acupuncture points, especially peripheral ones, have a lower skin resistance than the surrounding area. Instruments designed to measure skin resistance for the purpose of locating acupuncture points give acoustic or visual signals indicating points at which skin resistance is lowered. About 80 acupuncture points with reduced skin resistance can be accurately located with this method, most of them distal ones. Measurement of skin resistance is advisable for the beginner, and especially for the location of points on the ear. On the ear this method is of significant importance because areas there corresponding to disturbed organs or body regions develop reduced skin resistance. Therefore, this method is important as an additional diagnostic method for ear acupuncture.

Location with the Aid of Other Points

Examples:
Ex.6 Sishencong is located 1 cun in front of, lateral, and dorsal to Du 20 Baihui.
St.40 Fenglong and St.38 Tiaokou are located 5 cun below St.36 Zusanli.

Location of Painful, Sensitive, or Tender Points

These points are called Ah Shi points (locus dolendi) and are not necessarily classic acupuncture points. Needling of these sensitive or tender points is important in locomotor disorders.

4.4 Description of Channels and Points

4.4.1 Lung Channel   Lu.

Element: Metal
Coupled organ: Large intestine
Tissue: Skin
Sense organ: Nose, sense of smell
Maximal time: 3–5 a.m.
Alarm point, Mu: Lu.1 Zhongfu
Back Shu point: UB.13 Feishu (lateral to T3)

The lung channel is a Yin channel. The lung channel and the spleen channel together make up the **Tai-Yin axis.**

Course: The lung channel starts on the lateral side of the thorax in the 1st intercostal space, then descends along the radial side of the upper arm, along the radial side of the forearm to the wrist joint, and ends on the radial corner of the thumb nail.

Clinical applications: Treatment of respiratory disorders, disorders of throat and nose; skin disorders and painful disturbances along the channel.

Important points	Point categories, clinical applications
Lu.1 Zhongfu	Mu point, alarm point
Lu.5 Chize	He point, sedative point
Lu.6 Kongzui	Xi-cleft point
Lu.7 Lieque	Luo connecting point to LI.4 Hegu
	Confluent point for Ren Mai
Lu.9 Taiyuan	Yuan source point,
	tonification point,
	influential point for the vascular system

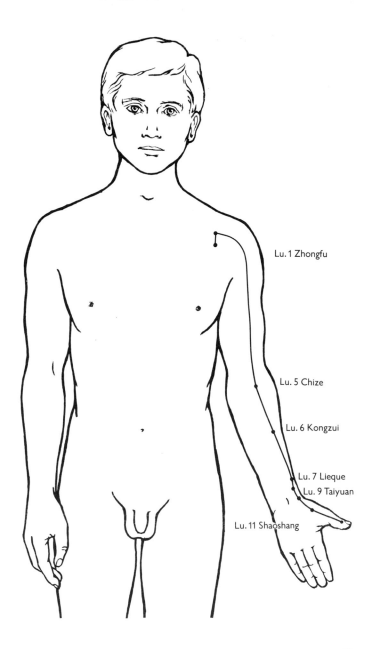

Lu. 1 Zhongfu

Lu. 5 Chize

Lu. 6 Kongzui

Lu. 7 Lieque
Lu. 9 Taiyuan

Lu. 11 Shaoshang

Lu.1 Zhongfu   Center of the prefecture   **Mu (alarm) point of the lung**

Location: On the lateral side of the anterior wall of the thorax in the 1st intercostal space. This point is located 6 cun lateral to the midline and in a relaxed shoulder girdle, 1 cun below the clavicle, below Lu.2 Yunmen.

Indications: As the alarm point of the lung this point is painful or tender on pressure in respiratory disorders. It is often used in disorders of the respiratory organs, such as bronchial asthma, bronchitis, bronchiectasis, and their symptoms, such as cough, dyspnea, and thorax pain.

Local point needling is performed here for pain in the shoulder girdle and pain on the lateral side of the thorax.

Needling method: Tangential and lateral, ca. 1 cm. Oblique direction to avoid injury of the pleura (pneumothorax).

Some acupuncture points are called **"dangerous" points** owing to their anatomical location, because dangerous injuries, e.g., pneumothorax can be caused by careless needling. Only carefull manual stimulation should be carried out at dangerous points.

Lu.5 Chize   Pond of the elbow   **He point, sedative point**

Location: At the elbow crease, lateral to the biceps tendon.

Indications: Arthritis of the elbow joint, lung disorders, paralysis of the arm. In psoriasis and other skin disorders, bleeding of this point may be effective. For this purpose relatively thick needles are used (0.5–1.0 mm). According to traditional medicine, the bleeding of points has an additional sedative effect for the vital energy. As a sedative point Lu.5 is used in lung and skin disorders according to traditional Chinese rules to sedate the excessive Qi. As a He point it corresponds to water and has a cooling effect.

Needling method: Perpendicular, 1–2 cm.

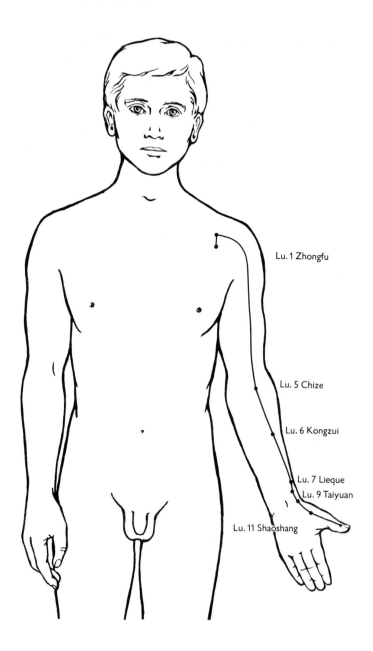

Lu. 1 Zhongfu

Lu. 5 Chize

Lu. 6 Kongzui

Lu. 7 Lieque

Lu. 9 Taiyuan

Lu. 11 Shaoshang

Lu. 7 Lieque   Mistake in row   **Luo connecting point to LI. 4, confluent point for Ren Mai**

Location: On the radial side of the forearm on the border of the radius, 1.5 cun proximal to the transverse crease of the wrist.

Indications: Disorders of the respiratory organs, such as bronchitis, common cold, bronchial asthma, bronchiectasis. Pain in the neck, back of the head, cervical spondylosis, tension and myogelosis of the neck muscles, headache, Parkinson's disease, skin disorders. Local disorders such as arthritis of the wrist or tendovaginitis. Lu. 7 Lieque is the most important point of the lung.

Lu. 7 Lieque is the Luo point of the lung channel, and therefore the starting point for the Luo vessel. The Luo vessel connects Lu. 7 Lieque with the coupled large intestine channel, at the Yuan point LI. 4 Hegu. Consequently, disturbances along the large intestine channel, e. g., rhinitis, toothache and facial paralysis, can be treated with Lu. 7 Lieque.

The course of the longitudinal Luo vessel leads to the lung and directly influences this organ. Therefore, this point is very important in the treatment of lung disorders.

Traditional application: Eliminates pathogenic factors especially cold, or heat and wind. It opens the surface of the body and has a strong dispersing function.

Needling method: Oblique, 1–2 cm.

Lu. 9 Taiyuan   Large deep abyss   **Yuan source point from LI. 6, tonification point, influential point for blood vessels**

Location: On the radial side of the wrist joint crease, lateral to the radial artery.

Indications: Disorders of the respiratory organs; arteriosclerosis and further blood vessel disorders (influential point of blood vessels), wrist pain, polyneuropathy of the upper extremity.

According to traditional Chinese theory Lu. 9 Taiyuan is one of the eight influential points. Lu. 9 Taiyuan is the influential point

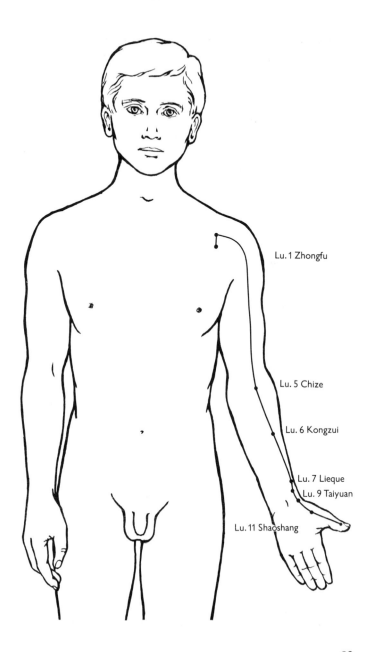

Lu. 1 Zhongfu

Lu. 5 Chize

Lu. 6 Kongzui

Lu. 7 Lieque

Lu. 9 Taiyuan

Lu. 11 Shaoshang

for disorders of the vessels, for example in arteriosclerosis, intermittent claudication, endarteritis, varicosis.

Lu.9 Taiyuan is the Yuan source point of the lung channel; this is where the Luo vessel, coming from the Luo point LI.6 of the large intestine channel, ends. It is also the tonification point of the channel. Tonification points, according to the traditional mother-and-son law, increase the energy of the corresponding organ. Moxibustion at tonification points has a very intense effect.

Needling method: Perpendicular, 0.5–1 cm.

Caution with needling: Avoid the radial artery.

Lu.11 Shaoshang Minor 2nd tone (Shang) **Jing well point**

The Chinese differentiate five tones (a pentatonic scale). The five tones are related to the five phases. The 2nd tone, Shang, corresponds to the element metal, and thus to the lung. The meaning is weak lung Qi.

Location: On the radial side of the thumb nail, ca. 3 mm proximal to the nail corner.

Indications: Treatment of acute emergencies such as fainting, collapse, epileptic attack, high fever, fever convulsions, cardiac and respiratory emergencies. Acupuncture should be combined with other emergency measures.

Jing well points are reserved for acute emergencies and other serious disorders, because needling is very painful.

Needling method: Perpendicular, 1–2 mm deep.

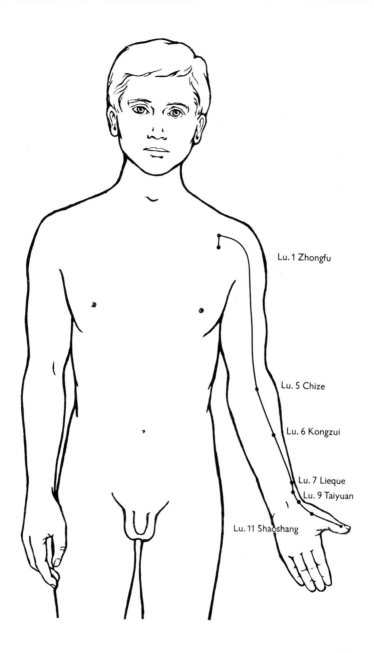

Lu. 1 Zhongfu

Lu. 5 Chize

Lu. 6 Kongzui

Lu. 7 Lieque
Lu. 9 Taiyuan

Lu. 11 Shaoshang

95

4.4.2 Large Intestine Channel LI.

Element: Metal
Coupled organ: Lung
Tissue: Skin
Sense organ: Nose, sense of smell
Maximal time: 5–7 a.m.
Alarm point, Mu: St.25 Tianshu (2 cun lateral to the navel)
Back Shu point: UB.25 Dachangshu (lateral to L4)

The large intestine channel is a Yang channel. The large intestine channel and the stomach channel together make up the **Yang-Ming axis.**

Course: The channel course runs from the radial corner of the index finger nail along the tabatière to the radial and dorsal side of the forearm, then to the radial side of the elbow crease. Along the lateral side of the upper arm it ascends to the shoulder, continues along the side of the neck to the face and ends lateral to the nose with LI.20 Yingxiang.

Clinical applications: The large intestine channel is coupled with the lung channel, and the two together constitute a functional unity; distal points of the large intestine channel are used in disorders of the related organ, the lung, and in skin disorders. Needling of large intestine points is also indicated in disorders along the channel course. **LI.4 Hegu** is the most important analgesic point in the body and is strongly stimulated in all painful conditions.
LI.11 Quchi, because of its homeostatic and immune-enhancing effects, is one of the most frequently used acupuncture points.

Important points	Point categories, clinical applications
LI.4 Hegu	Yuan source point from Lu.7
LI.11 Quchi	He point, tonification point

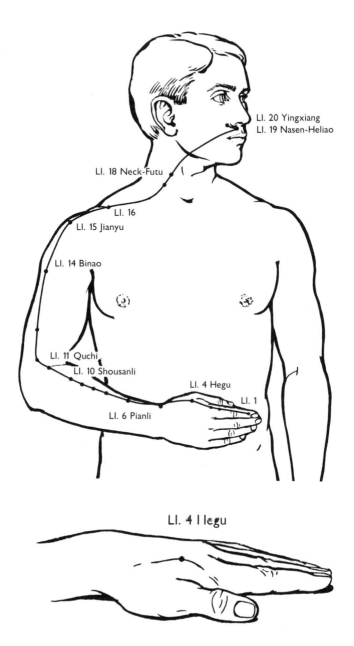

LI. 20 Yingxiang
LI. 19 Nasen-Heliao

LI. 18 Neck-Futu

LI. 16
LI. 15 Jianyu

LI. 14 Binao

LI. 11 Quchi
LI. 10 Shousanli

LI. 4 Hegu
LI. 1

LI. 6 Pianli

LI. 4 I Iegu

LI. 4 Hegu   Closed valley   **Yuan source point from Lu. 7**

Location: There are three possible ways of locating this important point:

1. At the highest point of the m. adductor pollicis with the thumb and index finger adducted. This method is the one most often used.
2. At the midpoint of the line bisecting the angle between the 1st and 2nd metacarpal bones when the thumb is fully extended.
3. Same level on the radial side of the 2nd metacarpal bone, above the 1st m. interosseus. This location is different from the first and second and is often used for acupuncture anesthesia.

Indications:
- Painful conditions; stimulation of this point relieves pain in all parts of the body.
- *LI. 4 Hegu is the most important analgesic point.*
- Treatment of disorders of the head area, especially of the face, the neck, and the teeth; common cold, sweating, fever, abdominal pain, painfree childbirth.
- The specific effect on the head, especially in headache has been verified by clinical research.
- Needling and stimulation of this point, owing to its good analgesic effect, is always indicated in all forms of pain treatment.
- LI. 4 Hegu is one of the most frequently used acupuncture points.

Traditional application: Promotes the flow of Qi, especially in the upper part of the body, eliminates pathogenic factors i.e. wind, cold, dampness from the head and lungs.

Needling method: Perpendicular, 1–2 cm, directed toward Pe. 8 Laogong; strong manual stimulation of the point has a significant analgesic effect.

LI. 11 Quchi   Pond on the curve   **He point, tonification point**

Location: On the end of the lateral transverse elbow crease, when the forearm is flexed at a right angle to the upper arm. Also to be located on the transverse crease at the middle of the connection between the biceps tendon and the lateral epicondylus of the humerus.

Indications: Homeostatic and immune-enhancing point. Therefore, this point is often used in allergic and infectious disorders, further-

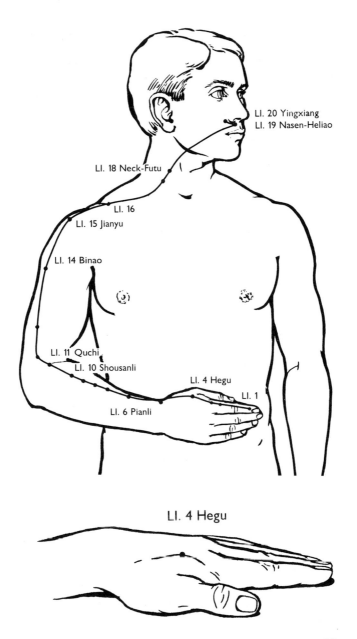

LI. 20 Yingxiang
LI. 19 Nasen-Heliao

LI. 18 Neck-Futu

LI. 16
LI. 15 Jianyu

LI. 14 Binao

LI. 11 Quchi
LI. 10 Shousanli

LI. 4 Hegu
LI. 1

LI. 6 Pianli

LI. 4 Hegu

more in skin disorders, endocrine disturbances, hypotension, hypertension, depression, states of weakness and as a local point in elbow disorders. LI.11 Quchi, because of its tonifying effect, is also very often heated with moxa in deficiency conditions.

Traditional application: Eliminates pathogenic factors especially heat and wind, it clears dampness and phlegm. Moxibustion of this point tonifies Qi and blood.

Needling method: Perpendicular, 2–3 cm.

LI.15 Jianyu   Shoulder clavicle

Location: With the arm abducted, on the shoulder in the anterior depression, palpable anterior to the tendon of m. biceps.

Indications: Periarthritis of the shoulder, paralysis of the arm, periarthritis humeroscapularis. Very important local point for the shoulder.

Needling method: Perpendicular, 1–2 cm.

LI.18 Neck Futu   Assistance for departure

Location: 3 cun lateral to the prominence of the thyroid cartilage, between the two bellies of m. sternocleidomastoideus.

Indications: Sore throat, cough, dysphagia, bronchial asthma, goiter.

Needling method: Perpendicular, 0.5 cm. A dangerous point.

LI.19 Nose Heliao   Small and long bone cleft

Location: Below the nose, 0.5 cun lateral from Du 26 Renzhong. Du 26 is located on the midline, on the border between the upper and middle third of the distance between nose and upper lip.

Indications: Rhinitis, common cold, nose bleeding, facial paralysis, trigeminal neuralgia, toothache.

Needling method: Oblique, 0.2–0.5 cm.

LI.20 Yingxiang   Welcome the smell

Location: Between ala nasi and nasolabial groove.

Indications: Rhinitis, blocked nose, common cold, nose bleeding, facial paralysis, trigeminal neuralgia, toothache. This point is often used together with Ex.1 Yintang in disorders of the nose. The most important distal point for this area is LI.4 Hegu and LI.11 Quchi.

Needling method: Oblique, 0.2–0.5 cm.

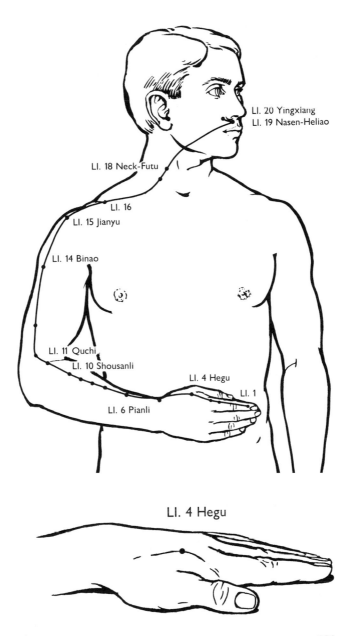

LI. 20 Yingxiang
LI. 19 Nasen-Heliao

LI. 18 Neck-Futu

LI. 16

LI. 15 Jianyu

LI. 14 Binao

LI. 11 Quchi

LI. 10 Shousanli

LI. 4 Hegu

LI. 1

LI. 6 Pianli

LI. 4 Hegu

4.4.3 Stomach Channel   St.

Element: Earth
Coupled organ: Spleen
Tissue: Connective tissue, "flesh"
Sense organ: Mouth
Maximal time: 7–9 a.m.
Alarm point, Mu: Ren 12 Zhongwan (middle navel and xiphoid)
Back Shu point: UB.21 Weishu (lateral to T12)

The stomach channel is a Yang channel. The stomach channel and the large intestine channel together make up the **Yang-Ming axis.**

Course: The stomach channel starts below the middle of the eye and courses in a U-turn to the temple. From St.5 Daying on the cheek the external branch runs downward along the throat to the fossa supraclavicularis. The channel follows the mamillary line along the thorax to the abdomen, where 2 cun lateral to the midline it continues on the anterior side of the thigh to the lateral side of the knee and lateral border of the tibia to the dorsum of the foot. The channel ends at the lateral corner of the 2nd toenail.

Clinical applications: The points of the face (St.1–8) are used in disorders of this area, e.g., eye disorders, migraine, facial paralysis, trigeminal neuralgia, and toothache. The points of the thoracic area are indicated in chest pain and in disorders of the mammary gland. Abdominal points (St.21, 25, 29) are selected in gastrointestinal disorders and in pelvic disorders. Points of the lower extremity

Important points	Point categories, clinical applications
St.1–8	Disorders of the face
St.21, 25, 29	Abdominal disorders
St.29 Guilai	Urogenital disorders
St.30, 36, 38, 41	Paralysis of the leg
St.36 Zusanli	He point, general tonification point
St.40 Fenglong	Luo connecting point to Sp.3
St.44 Neiting	Ying point, important analgesic point

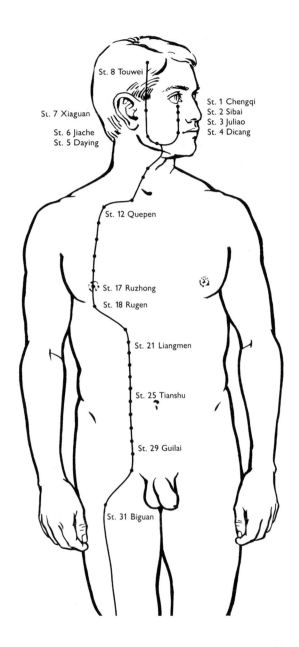

St. 8 Touwei

St. 1 Chengqi
St. 2 Sibai
St. 3 Juliao
St. 4 Dicang

St. 7 Xiaguan

St. 6 Jiache
St. 5 Daying

St. 12 Quepen

St. 17 Ruzhong

St. 18 Rugen

St. 21 Liangmen

St. 25 Tianshu

St. 29 Guilai

St. 31 Biguan

are used in the treatment of paralysis and joint disorders. Needling of points below the knee, as distal points, is indicated in abdominal disorders (St. 36, 40) and in disorders of the shoulder joint (St. 38) and of the face (St. 44).

St. 2 Sibai   Four white

Location: On the infraorbital foramen, 0.7 cun directly below St. 1 Chengqi. The first four stomach points are located on the vertical line below St. 1 Chengqi.
Indications: Trigeminal neuralgia, eye disorders, facial paralysis.
Needling method: Perpendicular, 0.2–0.5 cm.

St. 3 Juliao   Large bone cleft

Location: Directly below St. 2 Sibai at the level of the lower border of the ala nasi.
Indications: Trigeminal neuralgia, sinusitis, rhinitis, toothache, facial paralysis.
Needling method: Oblique or perpendicular, 0.5 cm.

St. 4 Dicang   Storage in the earth

Location: 0.5 cun lateral to the corner of the mouth, on the vertical line below the middle of the eyeball.
Indications: Trigeminal neuralgia, facial paralysis, hypersalivation, aphasia.
Needling method: Oblique, in lateral direction, 1 cm.

St. 5 Daying   Great welcome

Location: At the lowest point of the anterior border of the masseter muscle.
Indications: Trigeminal neuralgia, toothache, parotitis, facial paralysis.
Needling method: Perpendicular, 0.5 cm.

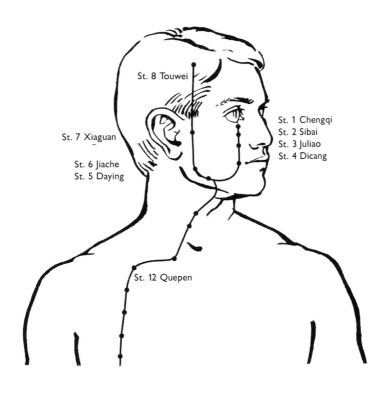

St. 8 Touwei

St. 7 Xiaguan

St. 6 Jiache
St. 5 Daying

St. 1 Chengqi
St. 2 Sibai
St. 3 Juliao
St. 4 Dicang

St. 12 Quepen

St. 6 Jiache   Cheek mechanism

Location: At the midpoint of the masseter muscle, when the jaw is closed.
Indications: Trigeminal neuralgia, toothache, parotitis, trismus, facial paralysis.
Needling method: Perpendicular, 0.5 cm.

St. 8 Touwei   Head binding

Location: 0.5 cun dorsal to the corner of the hairline on the forehead, just above St. 7 Xiaguan. This point is located 4.5 cun lateral to the midline and 3 cun above the level of the eyebrows.
Indications: Migraine, frontal and parietal headache, excessive lacrimation.
Needling method: Horizontal, 1 cm, posterior direction for headache, anterior direction for eye disorders. Most points of the scalp are needled in a tangential direction.

St. 21 Liangmen   Beam gate

Location: 2 cun lateral to the midline, 4 cun above the umbilicus. St. 21 is located lateral to Ren 12 Zhongwan, and the two points are often used together.
Indications: Acute and chronic gastritis, gastric and duodenal ulcer, gallbladder disorders, vomiting, nausea. This is an important local point for gastrointestinal disorders, often used together with Ren 12 Zhongwan.
Needling method: Perpendicular, 1–2 cm. A dangerous point.

St. 25 Tianshu   Celestial pivot   **Mu point of large intestine**

Location: 2 cun lateral to the umbilicus.
Indications: Acute and chronic gastroenteritis, diarrhea, constipation, vomiting, nausea, gastric and duodenal ulcers. As an alarm (Mu) point, important in diagnosis and treatment of disorders of the large intestine.
Needling method: Perpendicular, 1–2 cm. In weakness conditions, moxibustion of St. 21 Liangmen, St. 25 Tianshu and Ren 12 Zhongwan is indicated.

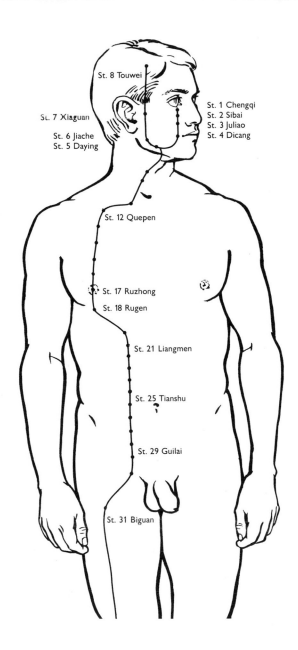

St. 29 Guilai   Coming back

Location: 4 cun directly below St. 25.
Indications: Constipation, diarrhea, irritable bowel disease, pelvic disorders, urogenital disorders, impotence.
Needling method: Perpendicular, 1–2 cm.

St. 35 Dubi   Calf's nose (also called Lateral **Xiyan**)

Location: In the depression lateral to the lower border of the patella when the knee is slightly bent.
Indications: Local point in painful disorders of the knee joint.
Needling method: Oblique towards the middle of the patella, 1–2 cm. On the medial side of the patella **Ex. 32 Xiyan** is located. The two points together are called calf's nose and are used together with **Ex. 31 Heding,** on the superficial border of the patella, as local points for treatment of knee joint disorders.

St. 36 Zusanli   Three units on the leg   **He point**

Location: One-finger's breadth lateral to the lower border of the tuberositas tibiae, 3 cun below the knee joint.
Indications:
- Most important distal point for abdominal disorders: gastritis, stomach and duodenal ulcer, vomiting, nausea, diarrhea, constipation.
- General tonification point in weakness conditions and hypotension.
- Homeostatic effects in diabetes mellitus and metabolic diseases, weakness and paralysis of the legs, and neuropathy.
- St. 36 Zusanli is one of the most effective acupuncture points, with a wide range of effects: spasmolytic and analgesic effect for the gastrointestinal tract, general tonification point, homeostatic effect in endocrine and metabolic diseases.
- Many scientific studies have verified the effectiveness of this point.

Traditional application: Tonifies the Qi and Yang, nourishes blood. It strengthens the defensive Qi (Wei Qi) and promotes the nourishment of internal organs.
Needling method: Perpendicular, 2–3 cm.

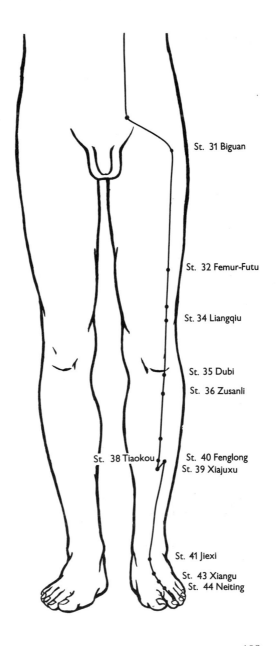

St. 31 Biguan

St. 32 Femur-Futu

St. 34 Liangqiu

St. 35 Dubi

St. 36 Zusanli

St. 38 Tiaokou

St. 40 Fenglong
St. 39 Xiajuxu

St. 41 Jiexi

St. 43 Xiangu
St. 44 Neiting

St. 38 Tiaokou Long opening

Location: 5 cun below St. 36 Zusanli, one-finger's breadth lateral to the anterior border of the tibia.
Indications: Frozen shoulder, periarthritis of the shoulder. St. 38 Tiaokou is highly specific as a distal point for the shoulder.
Needling method: Perpendicular, 2–3 cm, toward UB. 57 Chengshan. Manual stimulation to provoke a strong De Qi sensation.

St. 40 Fenglong Flourishing **Luo connecting point to Sp. 3**

Location: One-finger's breadth lateral to St. 38 Tiaokou, 2 cun lateral to the border of the tibia, 5 cun below St. 36 Zusanli.
Indications: Excessive sputum in bronchitis and bronchial asthma, epilepsy, fears, nuclear thinking, gastrointestinal disorders i. e., gastritis and ulcers.
Traditional application: Clears dampness and phlegm in the body, clears the Shen and eliminates heat from the stomach.
Needling method: Perpendicular, 2–3 cm.

St. 44 Neiting Interior hall **Ying point**

Location: 0.5 cun proximal to the margin of the web between the 2nd and 3rd metatarsal bones.
Indications: Important distal point for headache, toothache, abdominal pain, diarrhea. *Very important general analgesic point.*
Traditional application: St. 44 Neiting is eliminating heat and other pathogenic influences of the channel and promotes the flow of Qi.
Needling method: Perpendicular or oblique, 1 cm. Manuel or electrostimulation in severe pain and for anesthesia.

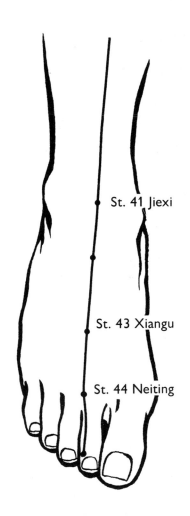

St. 41 Jiexi

St. 43 Xiangu

St. 44 Neiting

4.4.4 Spleen Channel   Sp.

Element: Earth
Coupled organ: Stomach
Tissue: Connective tissue, fatty tissue, "flesh"
Sense organ: Mouth
Maximal time: 9–11 a.m.
Alarm point, Mu: Liv.13 Zhangmen (11th rib)
Back Shu point: UB.20 Pishu (lateral to T11)

The spleen channel is a Yin channel. The spleen channel and the lung channel together make up the **Tai-Yin axis** (Tai Yin = Large Yin).

Course: The spleen channel starts on the medial side of the great toe nail, then runs along the medial side of the foot to the medial side of the leg and along here to the lateral side of the abdomen. It runs from the abdomen to the lateral and upper side of the thorax. It turns in a downward and lateral direction to end at the axillary line in the 6th intercostal space.

Clinical applications: According to traditional concepts the functions of the Chinese "spleen system" include the functions of the pancreas, i.e., the digestive function, and the functions of the spleen, with the immune system. The spleen system is traditionally believed to regulate water and blood metabolism, to influence the connective tissues, and to nourish the lips and tongue. Points of the spleen channel are indicated in disorders of the digestive system, urogenital disorders, and skin disorders.

Important points	Point categories, clinical application
Sp.3 Taibai	Yuan source point (of St.40)
Sp.4 Gongsun	Luo connecting point to St.42, confluent point of Chong Mai
Sp.6 Sanyinjiao	Junction of the three Yin channels: spleen, kidney, liver
Sp.9 Yinlingquan	He point
Sp.10 Xuehai	Immune-enhancing effect (sea of blood)
Sp.15 Daheng	Abdominal disorders

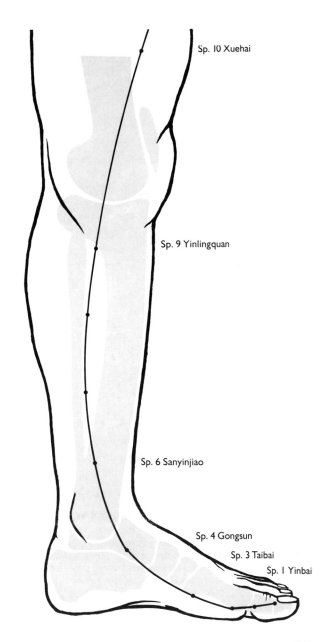

Sp. 10 Xuehai

Sp. 9 Yinlingquan

Sp. 6 Sanyinjiao

Sp. 4 Gongsun

Sp. 3 Taibai

Sp. I Yinbai

Sp. 3 Taibai   Great white   **Yuan source point from St. 40**

Location: Proximal to the head of the 1st metatarsal bone, on the medial side of the foot.
Indications: Pain in the upper abdomen, abdominal distention, diarrhea, vomiting, constipation.
Needling method: Perpendicular, 0.5–1 cm.

Sp. 4 Gongsun   Yellow emperor   **Luo connecting point to St. 42**

Location: In the depression distal to the base of the 1st metatarsal bone, on the medial side of the foot.
Indications: From this point a Luo vessel passes to the stomach channel; therefore Sp. 4 is indicated in stomach disorders, such as gastritis and dyspepsia, but also in diarrhea and constipation.
Needling method: Perpendicular, 1–2 cm.

Sp. 6 Sanyinjiao   Meeting of the three Yin
(San = 3, Yin = Yin channel, Jiao = junction)

Location: 3 cun above the medial malleolus, dorsal to the posterior border of the tibia.
Indications:
– Sp. 6 Sanyinjiao is one of the most important and most frequently used acupuncture points.
– Urogenital disorders and disturbances such as dysuria, frequent urination, retention of urine, impotence, prostatitis, dysmenorrhea, amenorrhea and pain in this area.
– Gastrointestinal disturbances such as diarrhea, maldigestion, abdominal distention.
– Important general tonification point for deficiency conditions i.e. chronic fatigue, depression, convalescence, and hypotension. Moxibustion is used here.
– Allergic and immunological disorders, endocrine disorders, such as diabetes mellitus; skin disorders.
– As Sanyinjiao is the meeting point of the three Yin channels (spleen, kidney, liver), Sp. 6 is also indicated in disorders of the kidney and liver.

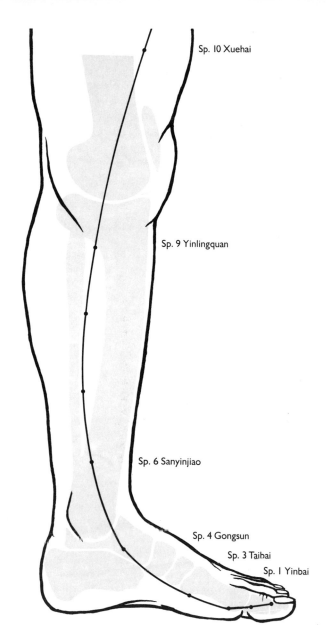

Sp. 10 Xuehai

Sp. 9 Yinlingquan

Sp. 6 Sanyinjiao

Sp. 4 Gongsun

Sp. 3 Taibai

Sp. 1 Yinbai

115

– For acupuncture anesthesia during surgical operations in the pelvic region and for analgesia during childbirth often combined with the extrapoint Neima.
– In childbirth these two points are electrostimulated.

Traditional application: Tonifies Qi in general but also spleen and stomach i.e. the middle Jiao. It nourishes the kidney Yin and tonifies the blood. Sp.6 Sanyinjiao as the meeting point of the lower 3 Yin promotes the spleen, kidney and liver organs. It clears damp especially from the lower part of the body.

Needling method: Perpendicular, 1–3 cm. Moxibustion is indicated in deficiency conditions.

Sp.9 Yinlingquan   Spring at the Yin grave hill   **He point**

Location: On the medial side of the leg, in the depression below the lower border of the medial condyle, at the level of the tuberositas tibiae.

Indications: Edema, ascites, and swelling of the lower extremities or of the kneejoint. Local point in painful conditions of this area.

Traditional application: Clears dampness.

Needling method: Perpendicular, 2–3 cm.

Sp.10 Xuehai   Sea of blood

Location: The highest point of the m.vastus medialis, 2 cun proximal to the upper border of the patella.

Indications: Important immune-enhancing point. Skin disorders, i.e. eczema, psoriasis, urticaria; allergies, infectious disorders, blood diseases, urogenital disorders.

Traditional application: Nourishes blood, promotes its flow and eliminates heat.

Needling method: Oblique, 2–3 cm.

Sp.15 Daheng   Large horizontal

Location: 4 cun lateral to the umbilicus, lateral to St.25.

Indications: Gastrointestinal disorders, diarrhea, constipation, gastritis, dyspepsia.

Needling method: Perpendicular, 2–3 cm.

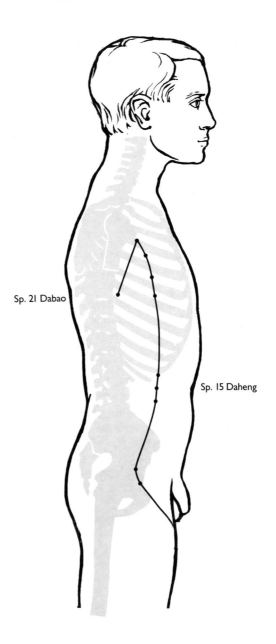

Sp. 21 Dabao

Sp. 15 Daheng

4.4.5 Heart Channel   He.

Element: Fire
Coupled organ: Small intestine
Tissue: Blood and blood vessels
Sense organ: Tongue
Maximal time: 11 a.m.–1 p.m.
Alarm point, Mu: Ren 14 Juque
Back Shu point: UB.15 Xinshu (lateral to T5)

The heart channel is a Yin channel. The heart channel and the small intestine channel together make up the **Shao-Yin axis.**

Course: The peripheral course descends from the axilla along the medial and ulnar side of the arm to the palm and ends on the radial side of the little finger at the nail corner.

Clinical applications: The heart, according to traditional Chinese theory, includes the function of the circulation besides the functions of the heart, and also the function of the brain, especially the consciousness. The activity of the mind and the emotional feelings are associated with the heart. Thus, points on the heart channel are psychologically effective. The heart "opens to the mouth" and thus determines the color of the tongue. According to the Chinese theory, the heart houses the shen, i.e., the spirit. The heart is the "emporer" governing all other organs.

Points on the heart channel are indicated in heart disorders, psychosomatic illness, psychological disorders such as insomnia, agitation, speech disturbances; furthermore, in mental disorders such as schizophrenia and epilepsy and in painful disorders along the channel, e.g., epicondylitis and tendovaginitis.

Important points	Point categories, clinical applications
He.5 Tongli	Luo connecting point to SI.4
He.6 Yinxi	Xi-cleft point
He.7 Shenmen	Yuan source point from SI.7, sedative point
He.9 Shaochong	Jing point, tonification point

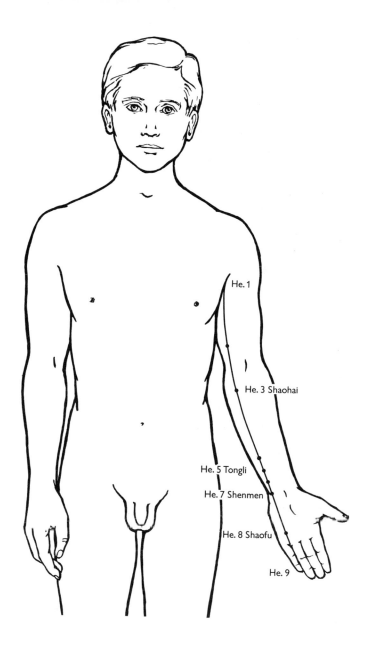

He. 1

He. 3 Shaohai

He. 5 Tongli

He. 7 Shenmen

He. 8 Shaofu

He. 9

He. 5 Tongli   Internal connection   **Luo connecting point to SI. 4**

Location: 1 cun proximal to He. 7 Shenmen, radial to the tendon of m. flexor carpi ulnaris.
Indications: Speech disturbances, aphasia, hoarseness, pain in the wrist, mental disturbances, vision disorders.
Needling method: Perpendicular, 0.5–1 cm.

He. 6 Yinxi   Yin cleft   **Xi-cleft point**

Location: 0.5 cun proximal to He. 7 Shenmen.
Indications: Acute angina pectoris, night sweating, acute cardiac disorders.
Needling method: Perpendicular, 0.5–1 cm.

He. 7 Shenmen   Gate of spirit   **Yuan source point from SI. 7, sedative point**

Location: On the transverse crease of the wrist, radial to the tendon of m. flexor carpi ulnaris. Needling is also possible from the ulnar side of the wrist, ulnar to the tendon of the m. flexor carpi ulnaris.
Indications: Mental disturbances, addiction, insomnia, anxiety states, epilepsy, chest pain, angina pectoris. Most important point for heart and mental disorders. This point is often used together with Pe. 6 Neiguan.
Traditional application: Calms the Shen and the heart (harmonizes the mind).
Needling method: Perpendicular, 0.5 cm. From the ulnar side, 1 cm.

He. 9 Shaochong   Minor impulse   **Jing well point, tonification point**

Location: On the radial side of the little finger, 2 mm proximal to the nail corner.
Indications: As a Jing point, in acute emergencies of heart and circulation, and in apoplexy and coma. Mental disturbances, fever, acute chest pain.
Needling method: Perpendicular, 1–2 mm.

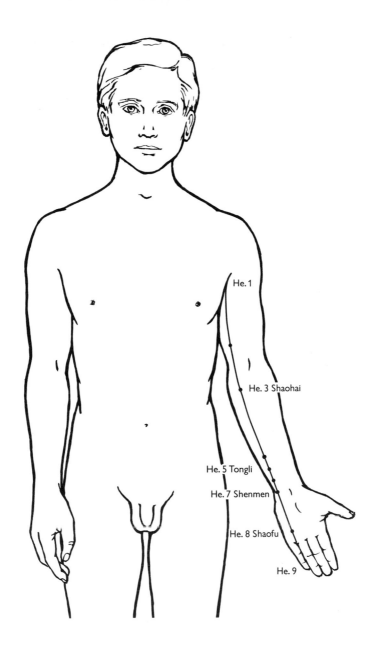

He. 1

He. 3 Shaohai

He. 5 Tongli

He. 7 Shenmen

He. 8 Shaofu

He. 9

4.4.6 Small Intestine Channel   SI.

Element: Fire
Coupled organ: Heart
Tissue: Blood and blood vessels
Sense organ: Tongue
Maximal time: 1–3 p.m.
Alarm point, Mu: Ren 4 Guanyuan
Back Shu point: UB.27 Xiaochangshu (lateral to S1)

The small intestine channel is a Yang channel. The small intestine channel and the urinary bladder channel together make up the **Tai-Yang axis.**

Course: The small intestine channel starts from the ulnar nail corner of the little finger and passes upward along the ulnar and dorsal side of the arm to the dorsal side of the shoulder. The channel runs along the shoulder in a zigzag line and continues on the lateral side of the neck and cheek to the ear.

Clinical applications: Treatment of painful disorders along the channel, e.g., epicondylitis, periarthritis of the shoulder, torticollis, cervical spondylosis, toothache, trigeminal neuralgia, ear disorders.

Important points	Point categories, clinical applications
SI.3 Houxi	Tonification point, confluent point of Du Mai, Shu point
SI.6 Yanglao	Xi-cleft point
SI.18 Quanliao	Trigeminal neuralgia

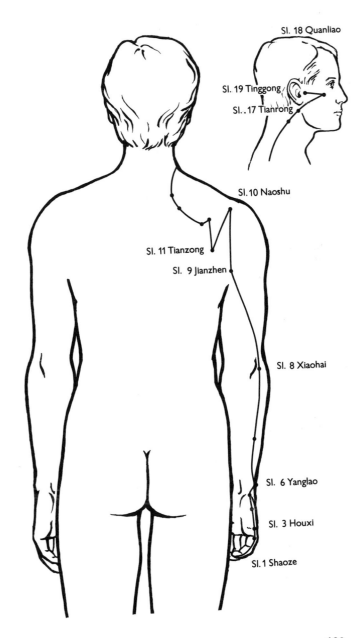

Sl. 18 Quanliao

Sl. 19 Tinggong

Sl. .17 Tianrong

Sl. 10 Naoshu

Sl. 11 Tianzong

Sl. 9 Jianzhen

Sl. 8 Xiaohai

Sl. 6 Yanglao

Sl. 3 Houxi

Sl. 1 Shaoze

SI. 3 Houxi Posterior brook **Tonification point, confluent point to Du Mai, Shu point**

Location: On the ulnar border of the hand with the fist clenched, at the ulnar end of the main transverse crease of the palm. This point is located proximal to the head of the os metacarpale toward the ulna.
Indications: Pain, tense muscles, and restricted movement of the neck and of the shoulder area, e.g., torticollis, cervical spondylosis. Important distal point in tinnitus, deafness, headache.
Traditional application: Eliminates pathogenic factors especially wind and dampness. It activates the Du Mai as its confluent point.
Needling method: Perpendicular, 1–2 cm, vigorous stimulation; this point may be painful.

SI. 6 Yanglao Age cherishing **Xi-cleft point**

Location: In the depression on the radial side of the styloid process of the ulna.
Indications: As a Xi-cleft point, in acute painful disorders along the channel, e.g., painful restricted movement of the neck or shoulder.
Needling method: Oblique, 1 cm, toward Pe. 6.

SI. 9 Jianzhen Steadfast shoulder

Location: When the arm is adducted, 1 cun above the dorsal crease of the axilla.
Indications: Periarthritis of the shoulder, paralysis of the arm.
Needling method: Perpendicular, 2–3 cm.

SI. 18 Quanliao Zygomatic bone cleft

Location: Caudal to the arcus zygomaticus, directly below the outer canthus of the eye.
Indications: Trigeminal neuralgia, sinusitis, toothache, facial paralysis.
Needling method: Perpendicular, 0.5–1 cm.

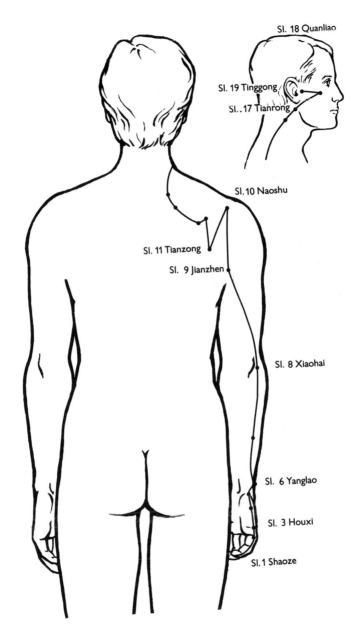

SI. 18 Quanliao

SI. 19 Tinggong

SI. 17 Tianrong

SI. 10 Naoshu

SI. 11 Tianzong

SI. 9 Jianzhen

SI. 8 Xiaohai

SI. 6 Yanglao

SI. 3 Houxi

SI. 1 Shaoze

125

4.4.7 Urinary Bladder Channel UB.

Element: Water
Coupled organ: Kidney
Tissue: Bones and joints
Sense organ: Ear
Maximal time: 3–5 p.m.
Alarm point, Mu: Ren 3 Zhongji
Back Shu point: UB.28 Pangguangshu (lateral to S2)

The urinary bladder channel is a Yang channel. The urinary bladder channel and the small intestine channel together make up the **Tai-Yang axis.**

Course: The urinary bladder channel starts from the inner canthus of the eye and ascends parallel to the midline over the forehead to the neck. At the neck the channel bifurcates into two branches; the more important medial branch descends 1.5 cun lateral and parallel along the midline to the level of the 4th sacral foramen, where it turns back upward to the 1st sacral foramen and then continues caudal to the dorsal side of the thigh to the hollow of the knee, to connect with the lateral branch. From the knee the channel descends along the dorsal side of the lower leg to the lateral aspect of the foot and ends on the lateral corner of little toe nail.

Clinical applications:
In disorders along the channel:

- Points on the face are used for eye disorders and for headache.
- Points on the neck are selected for occipital headache and cervical spondylosis.
- The Shu points on the medial branch are located segmentally. These paravertebrally located points have a direct influence on the segmentally corresponding internal organ. In acute and chronic disorders of the corresponding organs, the Back Shu points become tender on pressure or painful (Table 4.4).
- The points of the lumbar and sacral area are used for the treatment of kidney and urogenital disorders.
- The points located peripherally are indicated as distal points in lumbago, sciatica and urogenital disorders.

126

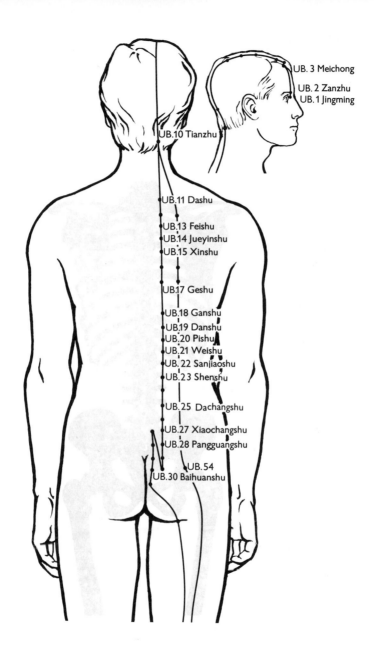

UB. 3 Meichong
UB. 2 Zanzhu
UB. 1 Jingming

UB.10 Tianzhu

UB.11 Dashu

UB.13 Feishu
UB.14 Jueyinshu
UB.15 Xinshu

UB.17 Geshu

UB.18 Ganshu
UB.19 Danshu
UB.20 Pishu
UB.21 Weishu
UB. 22 Sanjiaoshu
UB.23 Shenshu

UB. 25 Dachangshu

UB.27 Xiaochangshu
UB.28 Pangguangshu

UB. 54
UB.30 Baihuanshu

Important points	Point categories, clinical applications
UB.2 Zanzhu	Eye disorders, headache
UB.10 Tianzhu	Cervical spondylosis, occipital headache
UB.13 Feishu	Shu point of the lung (lateral to T3)
UB.15 Xinshu	Shu point of the heart (lateral to T5)
UB.17 Geshu	Shu point of the diaphragm (lateral to T7) influential point for blood
UB.18 Ganshu	Shu point of the liver (lateral to T9)
UB.19 Danshu	Shu point of the gallbladder (lateral to T10)
UB.20 Pishu	Shu point of the spleen (lateral to T11)
UB.21 Weishu	Shu point of the stomach (lateral to T12)
UB.23 Shenshu	Shu point of the kidney (lateral to L2)
UB.25 Dachangshu	Shu point of the large intestine (lateral to L4)
UB.27 Xiaochangshu	Shu point of the small intestine (lateral to S1)
UB.28 Pangguangshu	Shu point of the urinary bladder (lateral to S2)
UB.40 Weizhong	He point
UB.60 Kunlun	Jing point
UB.62 Shenmai	Psychologically effective

UB.2 Zanzhu   Covered with bamboo

Location: On the medial end of the eyebrow, directly above the inner canthus of the eye.
Indications: Eye disorders, frontal sinusitis, frontal headache, migraine.
Needling method: Perpendicular, 0.5–0.8 cm.

UB.10 Tianzhu   Celestial pillar

Location: 1.3 cun lateral to Du 15 Yamen (C1/2).
Indications: Headache, migraine, cervical spondylosis, common cold.
Needling method: Perpendicular or oblique, 0.5–1 cm.

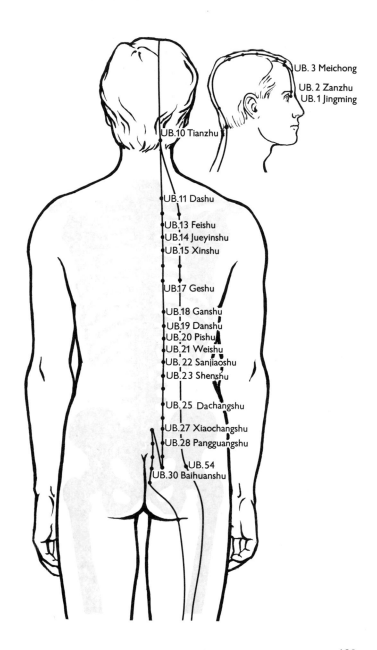

UB. 3 Meichong
UB. 2 Zanzhu
UB.1 Jingming

UB.10 Tianzhu

UB.11 Dashu

UB.13 Feishu
UB.14 Jueyinshu
UB.15 Xinshu

UB.17 Geshu

UB.18 Ganshu
UB.19 Danshu
UB.20 Pishu
UB.21 Weishu
UB. 22 Sanjiaoshu
UB.23 Shenshu

UB.25 Dachangshu

UB.27 Xiaochangshu
UB.28 Pangguangshu

UB.54
UB.30 Baihuanshu

UB. 13 Feishu   Transport point to the lung   **Shu point of the lung**

Location: 1.5 cun lateral to the lower border of the spinous process of T3.
Indications: Lung disorders, such as bronchial asthma, chronic bronchitis; also in cough and excessive sputum. The Shu points of the corresponding organ are often combined with the Mu or alarm points. In chronic lung disorders moxibustion of this Shu point is applied.
Needling method: Perpendicular, 1–2 cm.

UB. 15 Xinshu   Transport point to the heart   **Shu point of the heart**

Location: 1.5 cun lateral to the lower border of the spinous process of T5.
Indications: Heart diseases such as angina pectoris, mental disorders. Moxibustion of the points UB. 13–15 is often used in chronic disorders of the chest organs.
Needling method: Perpendicular, 1–2 cm. A dangerous point.

UB. 17 Geshu   Transport point to the diaphragm   **Shu point of the diaphragm, influential point for blood**

Location: 1.5 cun lateral to the spinous process of T7.
Indications: Hiccough, nausea, bronchial asthma, blood disorders.
Needling method: Perpendicular, 1–2 cm. A dangerous point.

UB. 18 Ganshu   Transport point to the liver   **Shu point of the liver**

Location: 1.5 cun lateral to the lower border of the spinous process of T9.
Indications: Liver and gallbladder disorders, eye disorders.
Needling method: Perpendicular, 1–2 cm. A dangerous point.

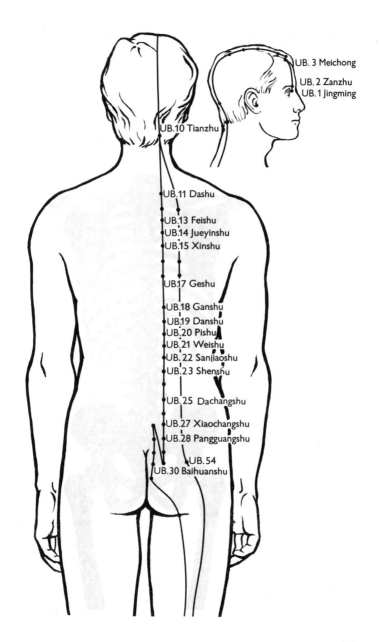

UB. 3 Meichong

UB. 2 Zanzhu

UB.1 Jingming

UB.10 Tianzhu

UB.11 Dashu

UB.13 Feishu

UB.14 Jueyinshu

UB.15 Xinshu

UB.17 Geshu

UB.18 Ganshu

UB.19 Danshu

UB.20 Pishu

UB.21 Weishu

UB. 22 Sanjiaoshu

UB.23 Shenshu

UB.25 Dachangshu

UB.27 Xiaochangshu

UB.28 Pangguangshu

UB. 54

UB.30 Baihuanshu

UB.19 Danshu Transport point to the gallbladder **Shu point of the gallbladder**

Location: 1.5 cun lateral to the lower border of the spinous process of T10.
Indications: Disorders of the gallbladder and biliary duct.
Needling method: Perpendicular, 1–2 cm.

UB.20 Pishu Transport point to the spleen **Shu point of the spleen**

Location: 1.5 cun lateral to the lower border of the spinous process of T11.
Indications: Digestive disorders, maldigestion, pain in the upper abdomen, diarrhea, pancreatic disorders.
Needling method: Perpendicular, 1–2 cm. A dangerous point.

UB.21 Weishu Transport point to the stomach **Shu point of the stomach**

Location: 1.5 cun lateral to the lower border of the spinous process of T12.
Indications: Gastric disorders such as ulcers and chronic gastritis.
Needling method: Perpendicular, 1–2 cm.

UB.23 Shenshu Transport point to the kidney **Shu point of the kidney**

Location: 1.5 cun lateral to the lower border of the spinous process of L2.
Indications: Urogenital disorders, dysmenorrhea, lumbago, sciatica, ear disorders. In deficiency conditions of the kidney, moxibustion is often applied.
Traditional application: Tonifies and nourishes the kidney Yin and Yang.
Needling method: Perpendicular, 1–2 cm.

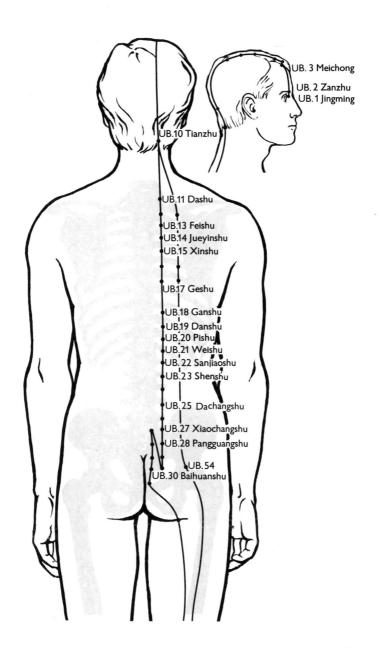

UB. 3 Meichong
UB. 2 Zanzhu
UB. 1 Jingming

UB.10 Tianzhu

UB.11 Dashu

UB.13 Feishu
UB.14 Jueyinshu
UB.15 Xinshu

UB.17 Geshu

UB.18 Ganshu
UB.19 Danshu
UB.20 Pishu
UB.21 Weishu
UB. 22 Sanjiaoshu
UB.23 Shenshu

UB. 25 Dachangshu

UB.27 Xiaochangshu
UB.28 Pangguangshu

UB. 54
UB.30 Baihuanshu

Table 4.4. Back Shu points with their functions

Points	Location	Name	Function	Translation
UB.13	**T3**	**Feishu**	**Shu of the lung**	Transport point to the lung
UB.14	**T4**	**Jueyinshu**	**Shu of the pericardium**	Transport point of the Yin
UB.15	**T5**	**Xinshu**	**Shu of the heart**	Transport point to the heart
UB.16	**T6**	**Dushu**	**Shu of the Du**	Transport point of the governing vessel (Du)
UB.17	**T7**	**Geshu**	**Shu of the diaphragm**	Transport point to the diaphragm, influential point for blood
UB.18	**T9**	**Ganshu**	**Shu of the liver**	Transport point to the liver
UB.19	**T10**	**Danshu**	**Shu of the gallbladder**	Transport point to the gallbladder
UB.20	**T11**	**Pishu**	**Shu of the spleen**	Transport point to the spleen
UB.21	**T12**	**Weishu**	**Shu of the stomach**	Transport point to the stomach
UB.22	**L1**	**Sanjiaoshu**	**Shu of the Sanjiao**	Transport point to the triple warmer
UB.23	**L2**	**Shenshu**	**Shu of the kidney**	Transport point to the kidney
UB.24	**L3**	**Qihaishu**		Transport point to the sea of vital energy
UB.25	**L4**	**Dachang-shu**	**Shu of the large intestine**	Transport point to the large intestine
UB.27	**S1**	**Xiaochang-shu**	**Shu of the small intestine**	Transport point to the small intestine
UB.28	**S2**	**Pang-guangshu**	**Shu of the urinary bladder**	Transport point to the urinary bladder

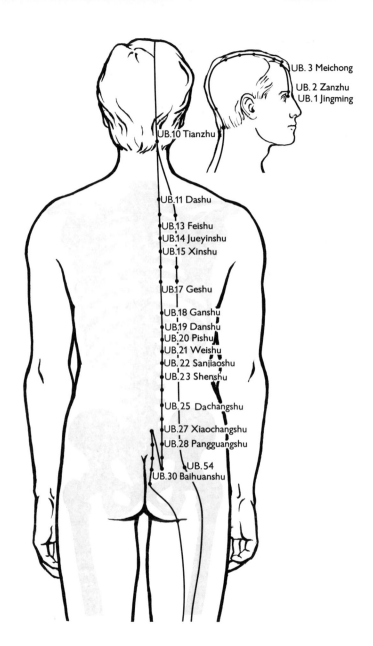

UB. 3 Meichong
UB. 2 Zanzhu
UB. 1 Jingming

UB.10 Tianzhu

UB.11 Dashu

UB.13 Feishu
UB.14 Jueyinshu
UB.15 Xinshu

UB.17 Geshu

UB.18 Ganshu
UB.19 Danshu
UB.20 Pishu
UB.21 Weishu
UB. 22 Sanjiaoshu
UB.23 Shenshu

UB.25 Dachangshu

UB.27 Xiaochangshu
UB.28 Pangguangshu

UB. 54
UB.30 Baihuanshu

UB.25 Dachangshu   Transport point to the large intestine   **Shu point of the large intestine**

Location: 1.5 cun lateral to the lower border of the spinous process of L4.
Indications: Diarrhea, constipation, abdominal distention, large intestine disorders, lumbago, sciatica.
Needling method: Perpendicular, 1–2 cm.

UB.27 Xiaochangshu   Transport point to the small intestine   **Shu point of the small intestine**

Location: 1.5 cun lateral to the midline, at the level of the S1 posterior foramen.
Indications: Intestinal disorders, urogenital disorders, lumbago, sciatica. In lumbago and sciatica the points UB.27–30 (S1 to S4) are needled. These points are also used with moxibustion.
Needling method: Perpendicular, 1 cm.

UB.28 Pangguangshu   Transport point to the urinary bladder   **Shu point of the urinary bladder**

Location: 1.5 cun lateral to the midline, at the level of the S2 posterior foramen.
Indications: Urogenital disorders, dysmenorrhea, lumbago, sciatica.
Needling method: Perpendicular, 1 cm.

UB.40 Weizhong   Center of the bend   **He point**

Location: At the midpoint of the popliteal transverse crease.
Indications: Lumbago, sciatica, pelvic disorders, impotence, enuresis. Very important point, often used together with UB.60 Kunlun.
Traditional application: Eliminates pathogenic factors especially wind and dampness but also heat from the blood. It promotes the flow in the channel therefore used mainly in low back pain.
Needling method: Perpendicular, 1–2 cm.

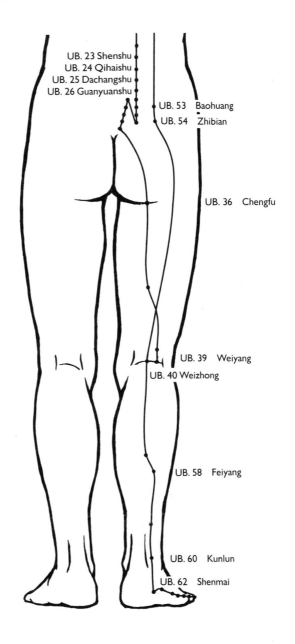

UB. 23 Shenshu
UB. 24 Qihaishu
UB. 25 Dachangshu
UB. 26 Guanyuanshu

UB. 53   Baohuang
UB. 54   Zhibian

UB. 36   Chengfu

UB. 39   Weiyang
UB. 40 Weizhong

UB. 58   Feiyang

UB. 60   Kunlun
UB. 62   Shenmai

UB. 60 Kunlun   Kunlun mountain   **Jing point**

The Kunlun mountain is regarded as supporting the heavens.

Location: At the middle of the connecting line drawn between the malleolus lateralis and the Achilles tendon.
Indications: Sciatica, lumbago, cervical spondylitis, distortions and pain of the ankle joint, tendinitis of the Achilles tendon, paralysis of the lower extremities.
Traditional application: Eliminates pathogenic factors i.e. wind and dampness. It promotes the flow in the channel.
Needling method: Perpendicular, 1–2 cm.

UB. 62 Shenmai   Announcing the pulse   **Confluent point for Yangqiao**

Location: 0.5 cun directly below the malleolus lateralis.
Indications: Mental disorders, convulsions, epilepsy, apoplexy, addictions, sleep disturbances.
Needling method: Perpendicular, 0.5–0.8 cm.

UB. 67 Zhiyin   Outer Yin   **Jing well point, tonification point**

Location: On the lateral side of the little toe, 2 mm proximal to the nail corner.
Indications: As Jing well point, for acute emergencies. Specifically indicated for analgesia in childbirth.
Needling method: Perpendicular, 1–2 mm.

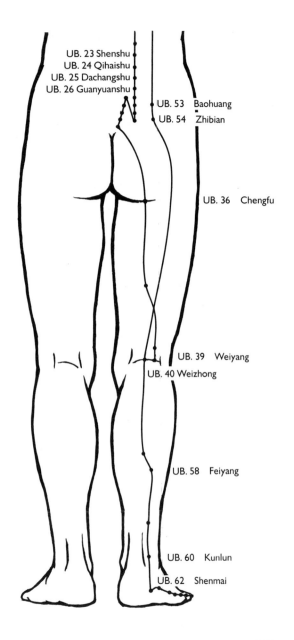

UB. 23 Shenshu
UB. 24 Qihaishu
UB. 25 Dachangshu
UB. 26 Guanyuanshu

UB. 53   Baohuang
UB. 54   Zhibian

UB. 36   Chengfu

UB. 39   Weiyang
UB. 40 Weizhong

UB. 58   Feiyang

UB. 60   Kunlun
UB. 62   Shenmai

4.4.8 Kidney Channel   Ki.

Element: Water
Coupled organ: Urinary bladder
Tissue: Bone
Sense organ: Ear
Maximal time: 5–7 p.m.
Alarm point, Mu: GB.25 Jingmen
Back Shu point: UB.23 Shenshu (lateral to L2)

The kidney channel is a Yin channel. The kidney channel and the heart channel together make up the **Shao-Yin axis.**

Course: The kidney channel originates on the sole of the foot. It runs to the medial side of the leg, then along to the abdomen, where the channel is located 0.5 cun lateral to the midline. In the thoracic area the distance from the midline is 2 cun. The channel ends in the depression below the clavicle.

Clinical applications: The kidney channel is coupled with the urinary bladder channel, and together they form a functional system. This includes the excretory function of the kidney and of the urinary tract and also the reproductive functions. The Chinese kidney system influences the willpower. Therefore deficiency of the kidney is relevant to a lack of willpower and thus also to mental depression.

The points on the kidney channel are mainly indicated in urogenital disorders, rheumatoid arthritis, and mental depression.

Important points	Point categories, clinical applications
Ki.3 Taixi	Yuan source point from UB.58
Ki.6 Zhaohai	Urogenital disorders
Ki.7 Fuliu	Jing point, tonification point

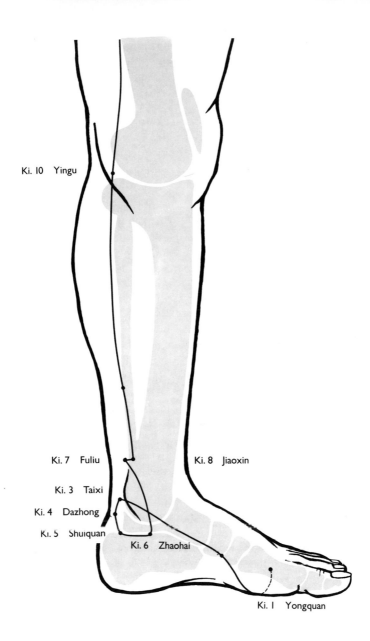

Ki. 10   Yingu

Ki. 7   Fuliu

Ki. 3   Taixi

Ki. 4   Dazhong

Ki. 5   Shuiquan

Ki. 8   Jiaoxin

Ki. 6   Zhaohai

Ki. 1   Yongquan

Ki. 3 Taixi   Large brook   **Yuan source point from UB. 58**

Location: Midway between the most prominent point of the malleolus medialis and the superior border of the Achilles tendon.
Indications: Urogenital disorders, enuresis, dysmenorrhea, impotence, cystitis, disorders of the ankle joint. Very important point for moxibustion in deficiency conditions.
Traditional application: Tonifies kidney Yin and Yang.
Needling method: Perpendicular, 1–2 cm.

Ki. 6 Zhaohai   Toward the sea

Location: 1 cun directly below the tip of the malleolus medialis.
Indications: Dysmenorrhea, amenorrhea, insomnia, anxiety restlessness, disorders of the ankle joint.
Traditional application: Tonifies especially kidney Yin neutralizes heat and calms the Shen and heart.
Needling method: Perpendicular, 0.5–1 cm.

Ki. 7 Fuliu   Reestablished flow   **Jing point, tonification point**

Location: On the anterior border of the Achilles tendon, 2 cun above the malleolus medialis.
Indications: Cystitis, nephritis, night sweats, diarrhea, lumbago; moxibustion in deficiency conditions.
Needling method: Perpendicular, 1–2 cm.

Ki. 8 Jiaoxin   Presents the message

Location: On the posterior border of the tibia, 2 cun above the malleolis medialis, 0.5 cun anterior to Ki. 7 Fuliu.
Indications: Kidney and urinary bladder disorders, moxibustion in deficiency conditions.
Needling method: Perpendicular, 1–2 cm.

Ki. 3 Taixi, Ki. 7 Fuliu, Ki. 8. Jiaoxin and Sp. 6 Sanyinjiao are often used for moxibustion in urogenital disorders with deficiency symptoms.

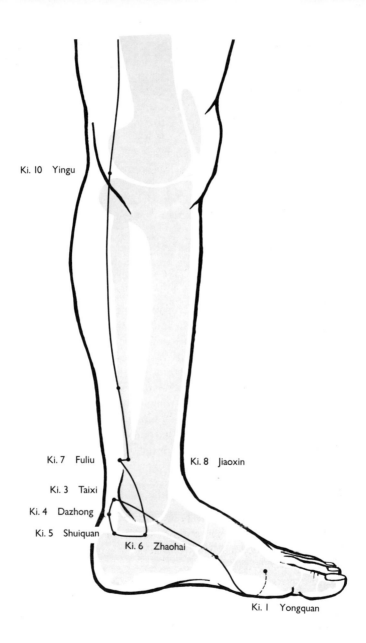

Ki. 10   Yingu

Ki. 7   Fuliu

Ki. 3   Taixi

Ki. 4   Dazhong

Ki. 5   Shuiquan

Ki. 6   Zhaohai

Ki. 8   Jiaoxin

Ki. 1   Yongquan

143

4.4.9 Pericardium Channel   Pe.

Element: Fire
Coupled organ: Sanjiao
Tissue: Blood and blood vessels
Sense organ: Tongue
Maximal time: 7–9 p.m.
Alarm point, Mu: Ren 17 Shanzhong
Back Shu point: UB.14 Jueyinshu (lateral to T4)

The pericardium channel is a Yin channel. The pericardium channel and the liver channel together make up the **Jue-Yin axis.**

Course: The channel starts lateral to the mamilla, then passes to the axilla, descending along the medial aspect of the arm to end at the tip of the middle finger.

Clinical applications: According to Chinese theory the heart and pericardium channels are associated with the brain and its functions. Heart and pericardium form a functional unit according to this idea, and this corresponds to the element fire. The pericardium is considered to protect and regulate the cardiac function. The heart is related more to the mental functions. Points of the pericardium channel have a strong effect on the circulation and are therefore indicated in cardiac and circulatory disorders.

Mental, psychosomatic, and gastroenterological disorders are the major indications for the points of the pericardium channel.

Important points	Point categories, clinical applications
Pe.4 Ximen	Xi-cleft point
Pe.6 Neiguan	Luo connecting point to SJ.4, confluent point Yinwei
Pe.7 Daling	Shu point, Yuan source point from SJ.5, sedative point

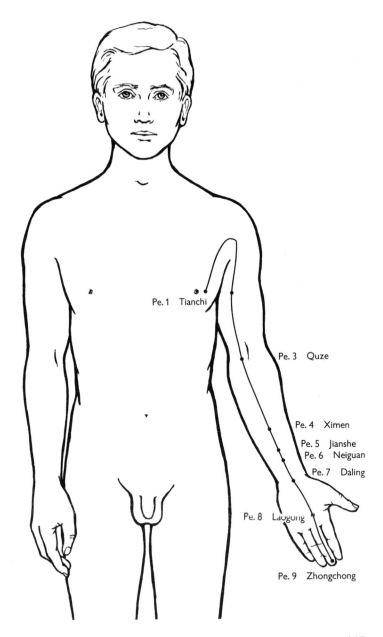

Pe. 1 Tianchi

Pe. 3 Quze

Pe. 4 Ximen

Pe. 5 Jianshe
Pe. 6 Neiguan
Pe. 7 Daling

Pe. 8 Laogong

Pe. 9 Zhongchong

Pe. 4 Ximen   Cleft gate   **Xi-cleft point**

Location: Between the tendons of m. palmaris longus and m. flexor carpi radialis, 5 cun proximal to the transverse crease of the wrist.

Indications: As Xi-cleft point, in acute disorders of the heart and circulatory system, such as angina pectoris, cardiac arrhythmia, tachycardia, pleuritis, mastitis, mental lability.

Needling method: Perpendicular, 1–2 cm.

Pe. 6 Neiguan   Inner pass   **Luo connecting point to SJ. 4, confluent point of Yinwei**

Location: Between the tendons m. palmaris longus and m. flexor carpi radialis, 2 cun proximal to the transverse crease of the wrist.

Indications:
- Heart disorders, disorders of the chest area (angina pectoris).
- Very important point in disorders of the upper abdomen (gastric and duodenal ulcers, gastritis, *nausea, hiccough, vomiting,* heartburn);
- Mental disorders and psychiatric diseases (vegetative dysregulation, restlessness, agitation, insomnia, epilepsy).

Traditional application: Regulates the flow of heart Qi and blood, clears the Shen and harmonizes the middle Jiao, especially the stomach.

Needling method: Perpendicular, 1–2 cm. For acupuncture anesthesia deep needling in the direction of SJ. 5 Waiguan.

Pe. 7 Daling   Big tomb   **Shu point, Yuan source point from SJ. 5, sedative point**

Location: On the transverse crease of the wrist, between the tendons of m. palmaris longus and m. flexor carpi radialis.

Indications: Wrist disorders, tendovaginitis, polyneuropathy, paralysis. Mental disturbances, schizophrenia, insomnia, epilepsy.

Needling method: Perpendicular, 0.5–1 cm.

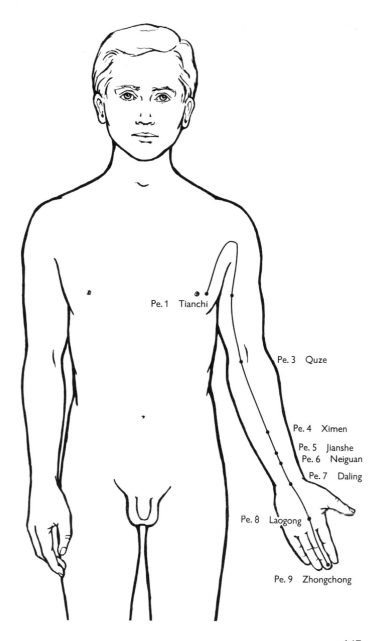

Pe. 1 Tianchi

Pe. 3 Quze

Pe. 4 Ximen

Pe. 5 Jianshe
Pe. 6 Neiguan

Pe. 7 Daling

Pe. 8 Laogong

Pe. 9 Zhongchong

147

4.4.10 Sanjiao Channel   SJ.

Element: Fire
Coupled organ: Pericardium
Tissue: Blood and blood vessels
Sense organ: Tongue
Maximal time: 9–11 p.m.
Alarm point, Mu: Ren 5 Shimen
Back Shu point: UB.22 Sanjiaoshu (lateral to L1)

The name of this channel is translated as "triple burner," "triple heater," or "triple warmer." The Sanjiao channel is a Yang channel. The Sanjiao channel and the gallbladder channel together make up the **Shao-Yang axis.**

Course: The Sanjiao channel starts on the ulnar corner of the nail of the ring finger, ascends along the dorsal side of the hand and arm to the shoulder, circles around the auricle, and runs to the lateral side of the eyebrow.

Clinical applications: The Sanjiao is a designation of functions of the organs in the three body cavities. The upper "warmer" is located in the chest controlling the lungs and the heart; the middle Jiao corresponds to the abdominal cavity and controls the digestive function, and the lower warmer is related to the pelvic region and rules excretion.

Important points	Point categories, clinical applications
SJ.3 Zhongzhu	Shu point, tonification point, distal point for ear disorders
SJ.5 Waiguan	Luo connecting point to Pe.7, important distal point for the head and neck
SJ.6 Zhigou	Jing point, for constipation
SJ.8 Sanyangluo	Connection of the three Yang channels, distal point for the chest wall
SJ.14 Jianliao	Disorders of the shoulder
SJ.17 Yifeng	Local point for ear disorders

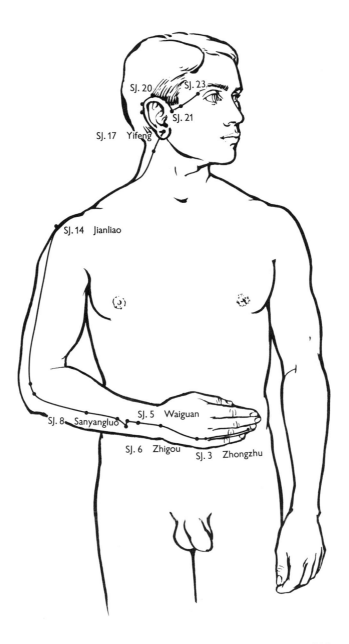

Points of the Sanjiao channel are selected:

- In deafness, tinnitus, dizziness
- In gastrointestinal disorders, such as constipation
- In chest and shoulder pain
- In headache and eye disorders

SJ.3 Zhongzhu   Center of the small island   **Shu point,
tonification point**

Location: On the back of the hand between the 4th and 5th metacarpal bones, proximal to the metacarpophalangeal joint.
Indications: Deafness, tinnitus, dizziness and other ear disorders, pain, paralysis, and polyneuropathies of the hands.
Needling method: Perpendicular, 1–2 cm.

SJ.5 Waiguan   Outer pass   **Luo connecting point to Pe.7**

Location: At the midpoint between ulna and radius, 2 cun proximal to the dorsal crease of the wrist.
Indications: Very important distal point in temporal headache, migraine, torticollis, common cold, fever, ear disorders; local point in paralysis, pain and polyneuropathy of the arm, arthritis of the wrist.
Traditional application: Eliminates pathogenic factors especially wind, cold or heat.
Needling method: Perpendicular, 1–2 cm.

SJ.6 Zhigou   Lateral groove   **Jing point**

Location: Between ulna and radius, 3 cun proximal to the wrist.
Indications: Constipation, irritable bowel disease.
Needling method: Perpendicular, 1–2 cm.

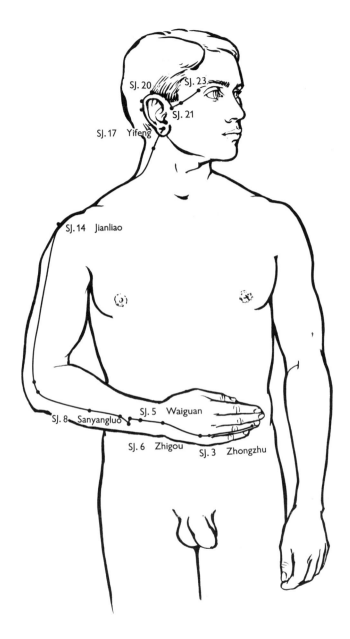

SJ. 20
SJ. 23
SJ. 21
SJ. 17 Yifeng
SJ. 14 Jianliao
SJ. 5 Waiguan
SJ. 8 Sanyangluo
SJ. 6 Zhigou
SJ. 3 Zhongzhu

SJ.8 Sanyangluo   Connection of the three Yang channels

Location: Between ulna and radius, 4 cun proximal to the wrist.
Indications: Distal point for pain in the chest wall, intercostal neuralgia, herpes zoster.
Needling method: Perpendicular, 1–2 cm.

SJ.14 Jianliao   Shoulder bone cleft

Location: In the more dorsally situated of the two depressions palpable on the shoulder when the arm is abducted.
Indications: Painful disorders of the shoulder, paralysis of the arm.
Needling method: Perpendicular, 1–2 cm, in direction of He.1 Jiquan.

SJ.17 Yifeng   Curtain in the wind

Location: In the depression posterior to the ear lobe, anterior to the mastoid process.
Indications: Deafness, tinnitus, dizziness, otitis media, parotitis, facial paralysis.
Needling method: Perpendicular, 1–2 cm.

SJ.21 Ermen   Gate of the ear

Location: When the mouth is opened, in the depression anterior to the intertragic notch, above the condyloid process of the mandible.
Indications: Deafness, tinnitus, dizziness, disorders of the mandibular joint.
Needling method: Perpendicular, 1–2 cm, with the mouth slightly open.

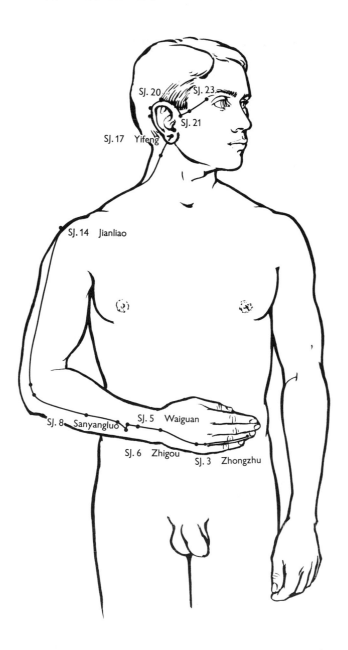

SJ. 20   SJ. 23

SJ. 21

SJ. 17   Yifeng

SJ. 14   Jianliao

SJ. 5   Waiguan

SJ. 8   Sanyangluo

SJ. 6   Zhigou

SJ. 3   Zhongzhu

4.4.11 Gallbladder Channel   GB.

Element: Wood
Coupled organ: Liver
Tissue: Muscle and tendon
Sense organ: Eye
Maximal time: 11 p.m.–1 a.m.
Alarm point, Mu: GB.24 Riyue (7th intercostal space)
Back Shu point: UB.19 Danshu (lateral to T10)

The gallbladder channel is a Yang channel. The gallbladder channel and the Sanjiao channel together make up the **Shao-Yang axis.**

Course: The gallbladder channel originates from the outer canthus of the eye and runs to the ear, circling around it and then curving downward to the occipital region. From here the channel runs back to the forehead and then returns backward parallel to the midline to the neck, passing further along the shoulder to the side of the chest and descending on the lateral side of the trunk along the lateral side of the abdomen, leg, and foot.

Important points	Point categories, clinical applications
GB.1 Tongziliao	Eye disorders
GB.2 Tinghui	Ear disorders
GB.14 Yangbai	Migraine, frontal headache
GB.20 Fengchi	Cervical spondylosis; occipital headache
GB.21 Jianjing	Additional alarm point of the gallbladder
GB.24 Riyue	Alarm point, Mu point of the gallbladder
GB.25 Jingmen	Alarm point, Mu point of the kidney
GB.30 Huantiao	Sciatica
GB.34 Yanglingquan	He point, influential point for muscles and tendons
GB.37 Guangming	Luo connecting point to Liv.3
GB.39 Xuanzhong	Influential point for marrow
GB.40 Qiuxu	Yuan source point from Liv.5
GB.41 Foot Linqi	Confluent point of Dai Mai, Shu point

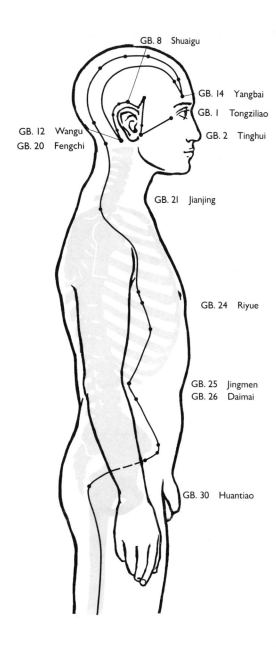

GB. 8 Shuaigu

GB. 14 Yangbai

GB. 1 Tongziliao

GB. 2 Tinghui

GB. 12 Wangu

GB. 20 Fengchi

GB. 21 Jianjing

GB. 24 Riyue

GB. 25 Jingmen
GB. 26 Daimai

GB. 30 Huantiao

155

Clinical applications: The gallbladder channel is closely related functionally to the liver. Both channels influence the metabolic functions and, according to traditional theory, are responsible for the flow of the vital energy, Qi. Needling of points on the gallbladder channel in the trunk region and of important distal points is indicated in liver and gallbladder disorders, low back pain, sciatica, paralysis, and disorders of the breast. Points on the head and in the neck area are used in eye and ear disorders, headache, migraine, and for cervical spondylosis.

GB.1 Tongziliao   Pupillar bone cleft

Location: 0.5 cun lateral to the outer canthus of the eye.
Indications: Eye disorders, frontal and occipital headache, trigeminal neuralgia.
Needling method: Oblique, 1–2 cm in lateral direction.

GB.2 Tinghui   Can hear

Location: When the mouth is opened, the point is palpable in a depression behind the condyle of the mandible.
Indications: Deafness, tinnitus, dizziness, otitis.
Needling method: Perpendicular, 1–2 cm.

GB.14 Yangbai   White Yang

Location: On the forehead 1 cun above the midpoint of the eyebrow.
Indications: Eye disorders, headache, migraine, trigeminal neuralgia.
Needling method: Oblique, 0.5–1 cm.

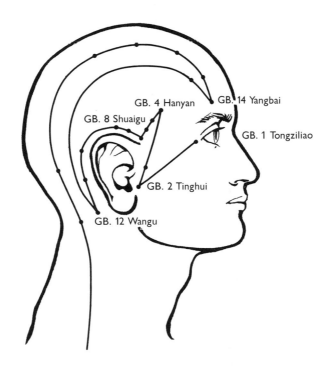

GB. 20 Fengchi   Wind pond

Location: Between the origins of m. sternocleidomastoid and m. trapezius.
Indications: Torticollis, cervical spondylosis, occipital headache, common cold, dizziness, hypertension.
Needling method: Perpendicular, 1 cm.

GB. 21 Jianjing   Shoulder well   **Additional alarm point of the gallbladder**

Location: At the highest point on the shoulder between the prominence (Du 14 Dazhui) and the acromion.
Indications: Gallbladder and liver disorders, periarthritis of the shoulder, myogelosis.
Needling method: Perpendicular, 1–2 cm. A dangerous point.

GB. 24 Riyue   Sun and moon   **Mu point of the gallbladder**

Location: On the mamillary line in the 7th intercostal space.
Indications: Liver disorders, hepatitis, cholecystitis, gastritis, hiccough.
Needling method: Oblique, 1–2 cm. A dangerous point.

GB. 25 Jingmen   Gate of the capital   **Mu point of the kidney**

Location: At the lower border of the free end of the 12th rib.
Indications: Disorders of liver and gallbladder, intercostal neuralgia. In kidney disorders together with UB. 23 Shenshu, the Shu point of the kidney. Moxibustion of both points is often used in deficiency conditions of the kidney.
Needling method: Perpendicular, 0.5–1 cm.

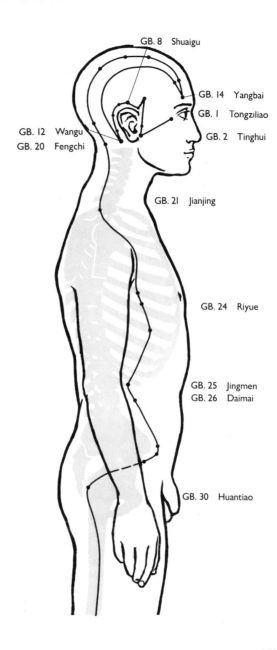

GB. 8   Shuaigu

GB. 14   Yangbai

GB. 1   Tongziliao

GB. 2   Tinghui

GB. 12   Wangu

GB. 20   Fengchi

GB. 21   Jianjing

GB. 24   Riyue

GB. 25   Jingmen

GB. 26   Daimai

GB. 30   Huantiao

GB. 26 Daimai   Belt vessel

Location: Midway between the free ends of the 11th and 12th ribs, at the level of the navel.
Indications: Disorders of liver and gallbladder, lumbago, backache, menstrual disorders, cystitis, bowel disease, feeling of distention in the abdomen.
Needling method: Perpendicular, 1–3 cm.

GB. 30 Huantiao   Jump in circles

Location: On the line from the trochanter major to the lower border of the sacral bone, at the border between the outer and middle thirds of this distance.
Indications: Sciatica, low back pain, coxarthrosis, paralysis, and polyneuropathy of the leg.
Needling method: Perpendicular, 4–8 cm.

GB. 34 Yanglingquan   Yang grave spring   **He point, influential point for muscles and tendons**

Location: At the point of intersection of the lines from the anterior and inferior borders to the head of the fibula.
Indications: This is a very important point. As an influential point in disorders of muscles and tendons such as rheumatoid arthritis, tendovaginitis, myopathy; intercostal neuralgia, liver and mental disorders, local point in disorders of the knee joint.
Traditional application: Promotes the flow of Qi, especially in stagnation of liver Qi. Eliminates pathogenic factors.
Needling method: Perpendicular, 2–3 cm. Also oblique, in downward and anterior direction.

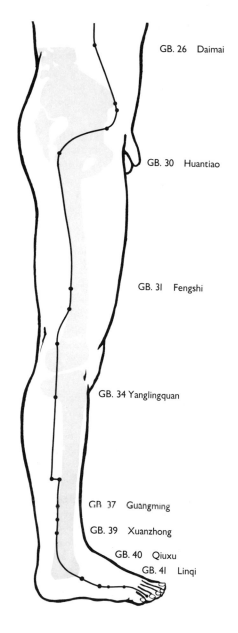

GB. 26   Daimai

GB. 30   Huantiao

GB. 31   Fengshi

GB. 34 Yanglingquan

GB. 37   Guāngming

GB. 39   Xuanzhong

GB. 40   Qiuxu

GB. 4I   Linqi

GB. 37 Guangming   Bright light   **Luo connecting point to Liv. 3**

Location: On the anterior side of the fibula, 5 cun proximal to the malleolus lateralis.
Indications: Eye disorders, headache, mental disorders.
Disorders of the coupled organs, liver and gallbladder, lactation disorders.
Traditional application: Promotes the flow of liver Qi, eliminates wind and dampness, clears the vision.
Needling method: Perpendicular, 1–3 cm.

GB. 39 Xuanzhong   Hanging of the bell   **Influential point for marrow**

Location: Between the posterior border of the fibula and the tendons of m. peroneus longus and brevis, 3 cun proximal to the malleolus lateralis.
Indications: Important distal point for torticollis and cervical spondylitis. As an influential point for the marrow in blood disorders.
Needling method: Perpendicular, 1–2 cm.

GB. 40 Qiuxu   Barre hill   **Yuan source point from Liv. 5**

Location: Anterior and inferior to the malleolus lateralis; at the intersection of the line drawn from anterior and inferior malleoli laterale.
Indications: Arthritis, distortion of the ankle joint, lower leg ulcers, distal point in chest pain and mastitis.
Needling method: Perpendicular, 0.5–1 cm.

GB. 41 Foot Linqi   On the foot nearly weeping   **Confluent point of Dai Mai, Shu point**

Location: Distal to the base of the 4th and 5th metatarsal bones.
Indications: Important distal point for deafness, tinnitus, Ménière's syndrome, mastitis, locomotor disorders and dysmenorrhea.
Needling method: Perpendicular, 1–2 cm.

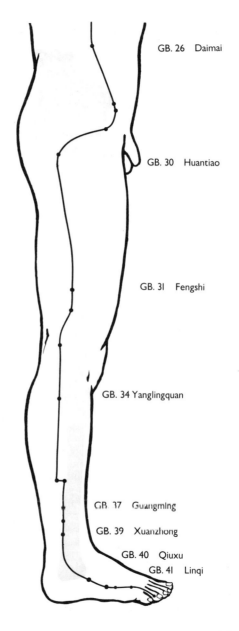

GB. 26   Daimai

GB. 30   Huantiao

GB. 31   Fengshi

GB. 34 Yanglingquan

GB. 37   Guangming

GB. 39   Xuanzhong

GB. 40   Qiuxu

GB. 41   Linqi

163

4.4.12 Liver Channel   Liv.

Element: Wood
Coupled organ: Gallbladder
Tissue: Muscle and tendon
Sense organ: Eye
Maximal time: 1–3 a.m.
Alarm point, Mu: Liv.14 Qimen
Back Shu point: UB.18 Ganshu (lateral to T9)

The liver channel is a Yin channel. The liver channel and the pericardium channel together make up the **Jue-Yin axis.**

Course: The liver channel runs from the great toe along the medial side of the leg and thigh to the external genitalia, then ascends to the abdomen, to end at the lateral chest wall in the 6th intercostal space below the mamilla.

Clinical applications: The liver channel is closely related to the genitals and also to the eye. The distal points of the liver channel are indicated in disturbances of the urogenital functions, metabolic disorders, liver and gallbladder disorders, eye disorders and headache. Points on the trunk are used in hepatic, cholecystic, and metabolic disorders.

Important points	Point categories, clinical applications
Liv.3 Taichong	Yuan source point from GB.37
Liv.8 Ququan	He point, tonification point
Liv.13 Zhangmen	Mu point of the spleen, influential point of the Zang organs
Liv.14 Qimen	Mu point of the liver

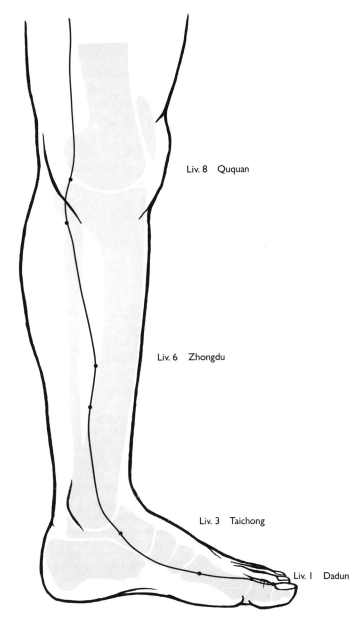

Liv. 8   Ququan

Liv. 6   Zhongdu

Liv. 3   Taichong

Liv. I   Dadun

Liv. 3 Taichong   Large impulse   **Yuan source point from GB. 37**

Location: Between the 1st and 2nd metatarsal bones, 2 cun proximal to the margin of the web.
Indications: Very important point in liver and gallbladder disorders, migraine, hypertension. Distal point for eye disorders, pain of the head and chest, urogenital, endocrine and metabolic disorders. In mental disorders and in stagnation of the flow of Qi. Liv. 3 and LI. 4 Hegu are often used together.
Traditional application: Promotes the flow of Qi, especially in the liver. It harmonizes liver excess conditions, eliminates wind and other pathogenic factors and calms the Shen.
Needling method: Perpendicular, 1–2 cm.

Liv. 8 Ququan   Spring in the curve   **He point, tonification point**

Location: At the medial end of the transverse popliteal crease, at the anterior border of m. semimembranosus and m. semitendinosus.
Indications: Urogenital infections, impotence, dysmenorrhea, disorders of the knee joint; moxibustion.
Needling method: Perpendicular, 2–3 cm.

Liv. 13 Zhangmen   Item gate   **Mu point of the spleen, influential point of Zang organs**

Location: At the free end of the 11th rib.
Indications: Disorders of liver and gallbladder, metabolic disorders; influential point of Zang organs (lung, heart, spleen, kidney, liver).
Needling method: Perpendicular, 1–2 cm.

Liv. 14 Qimen   Last gate   **Mu point of the liver**

Location: On the mamillary line in the 6th intercostal space.
Indications: Liver disorders, pain of the upper abdomen and chest, heart disorders, bronchial asthma, intercostal neuralgia, mastitis, lactation disorders.
Needling method: Oblique, 1–2 cm. A dangerous point.

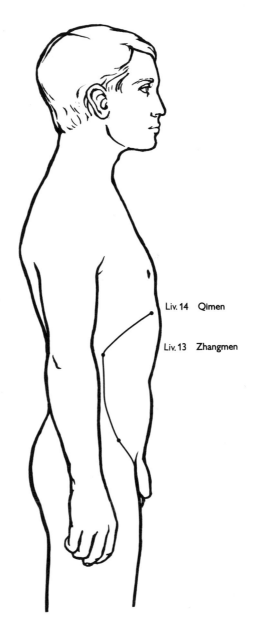

Liv. 14   Qimen

Liv. 13   Zhangmen

4.4.13 Du Mai

Du Mai (Wade-Giles: *Tou Mo*) means **governing vessel (GV.)**. The Du Mai and the Ren Mai channels are classed among the eight "extraordinary channels," *Qi Jingba Mai*. No internal organ is related to the Du Mai channel, but it is closely related to the central nervous system. The Du Mai is considered to be the governor of the six Yang channels, with an important controlling and governing role.

Course: The Du Mai starts at the os coccygis and passes upward along the dorsal midline to the neck, then runs along the midline of the head to the forehead and nose, to end below the upper lip in the mouth.

Clinical applications: Governing the six Yang channels, the Du Mai has an important coordinating and harmonizing effect on all regions of the body and all organs:
- Points in the lumbar and sacral region are indicated in urogenital disorders and in lumbago.
- Points in the chest and neck regions are selected in chest pain, cervical spondylosis, intercostal neuralgia, immune deficiency, fever and infectious disorders.
- Points on the cranial course are important in mental, psychosomatic and neurologic disorders, and in headache and migraine.
- The point Du 20 Baihui, located on the vertex of the skull, is the most important governing and harmonizing point and is therefore indicated for every acupuncture treatment.

Du 4 Mingmen   Gate of life   **L2/3**

Location: Between the spinous processes of L2 and L3.
Indications: Lumbago, sciatica, urogenital disorders.
Traditional application: Tonifies kidney Yang and the fire of the gate of life (Mingmen).
Needling method: Perpendicular, 1 cm.

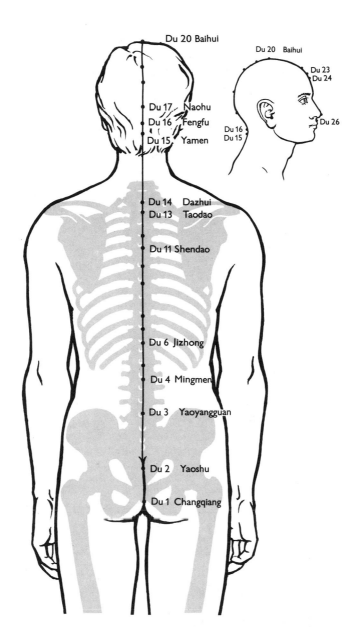

Du 20 Baihui

Du 20 Baihui
Du 23
Du 24

Du 17 Naohu
Du 16 Fengfu
Du 15 Yamen

Du 16
Du 15

Du 26

Du 14 Dazhui
Du 13 Taodao

Du 11 Shendao

Du 6 Jizhong

Du 4 Mingmen

Du 3 Yaoyangguan

Du 2 Yaoshu

Du 1 Changqiang

Du 6 Jizhong   Center of the spine   **T11/12**

Location: Below the spinous process of T11.
Indications: Lumbago, sciatica, intercostal neuralgia. In the treatment of spastic paralysis electrostimulation is also applied at Du 2 or Ex. 20.
Needling method: Oblique, 1 cm.

Du 11 Shendao   Way of the spirit   **T5/6**

Location: Below the spinous process of T5.
Indications: Weakness of memory, anxiety states, mental disorders, intercostal neuralgia.
Traditional application: Calms the Shen, promotes the heart Qi.
Needling method: Oblique, 1 cm.

Du 13 Taodao   Content way   **T1/2**

Location: Below the spinous process of T1.
Indications: Cervical spondylosis, occipital headache, fever, infectious disease.
Traditional application: Eliminates pathogenic influences, especially heat.
Needling method: Oblique, 1–2 cm.

Du 14 Dazhui   Large vertebra   **C7/T1**

Location: Below the spinous process of the vertebra prominens (C7).
Indications:
– Fever, infectious disease, immune-enhancing effect.
– Psychiatric disorders such as depression, schizophrenia.
– Bronchial asthma, eczema.
– Important point in occipital headache, cervical spondylosis, torticollis.
Traditional application: Eliminates pathogenic influences, especially heat and wind. Tonifies the Yang Qi and clears the Shen.
Needling method: Perpendicular, 1–2 cm.

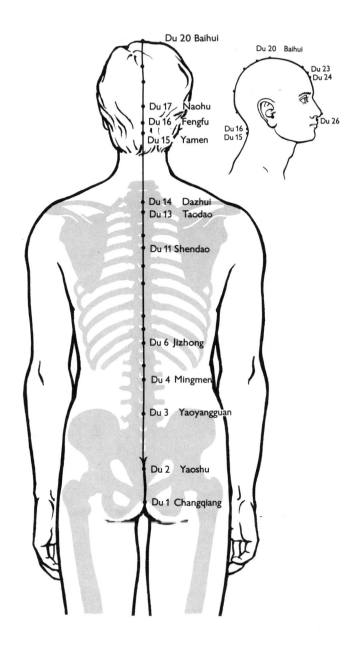

Du 20 Baihui

Du 20 Baihui
Du 23
Du 24
Du 26

Du 17 Naohu
Du 16 Fengfu
Du 15 Yamen

Du 16
Du 15

Du 14 Dazhui
Du 13 Taodao

Du 11 Shendao

Du 6 Jizhong

Du 4 Mingmen

Du 3 Yaoyangguan

Du 2 Yaoshu

Du 1 Changqiang

Du 20 Baihui   Hundred meetings

Location: On the continuation of the line connecting the lowest and highest points of the ear, on the median line of the head; 7 cun above the posterior hairline, 5 cun behind the anterior hairline.

Indications:
- Psychologically very effective point, general sedative and harmonizing effect.
- Very important point in headache, apoplexy, weakness of memory, distal point for anorectal disorders.
- This point can be used in every acupuncture treatment because of its general psychological and coordinating effect.
- Little stimulation by hand and no electrostimulation.
- This point is often used together with Ex. 6 Sishencong.

Traditional application: Promotes the *clear* Yang in the head, calms the Shen.

Needling method: Oblique, in posterior direction, 0.5 cm.

Du 26 Renzhong   Center of the upper lip

Location: At the border of the middle and upper thirds of the distance between nose and upper lip.

Indications: Du 26 is the Jing well point of the Du Mai, the most important Jing well point of the body. Specific in acute emergencies, such as collapse, shock, and epileptic attack.

It is the most important point in acute emergencies.

Epileptic attacks can be directly interrupted.

Needling method: Oblique in upward direction, 0.5 cm. Strong stimulation in epileptic attack. If no acupuncture needle is available, the nail of the index finger or a disposable cannula should be used.

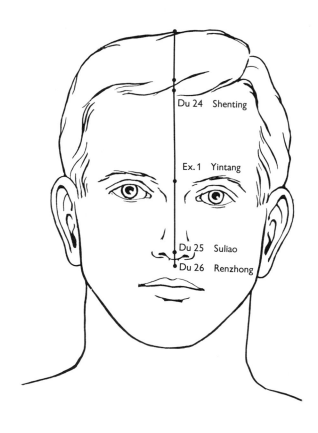

Du 24   Shenting

Ex. 1   Yintang

Du 25   Suliao

Du 26   Renzhong

4.4.14 Ren Mai

The Ren Mai (Wade-Giles: *Jenn Mo*) and the Du Mai channels do not correspond directly to an internal organ. The Ren Mai controls the six Yin channels and the five Zang organs. The Ren Mai influences the genital organs and is therefore called the **conceptional vessel (CV.)**.

Course: The Ren Mai channel starts from the perineum, ascending along the front midline over the abdomen and thorax to end below the mouth.

Clinical applications: The Ren Mai, controlling the six Yin channels, has a coordinating and harmonizing effect in disorders of the Yin organs, e.g., spleen, liver, kidney, lung, and heart. The points of the Ren Mai are therefore often indicated in urogenital, in gastrointestinal disorders and in disorders of the heart and lung. The Ren Mai is the site of many alarm points: Ren 12 Zhongwan, the alarm point of the stomach; Ren 14 Juque, that of the heart; and Ren 17 Shanzhong, that of the pericardium. There are also many tonification points on the Ren Mai channel, such as Ren 6 Qihai, sea of vital energy, and Ren 8 Shenque, the navel (only for moxibustion, not to be needled).

Ren 3 Zhongji   in the middle between the poles   **Mu point of the urinary bladder**

Location: On the midline, 1 cun above the symphysis.
Indications: Urogenital disorders, dysmenorrhea, cystitis, enuresis. Important for moxibustion.
Needling method: Perpendicular, 2–3 cm.

Ren 4 Guanyuan   Surrounded source energy   **Mu point of the small intestine**

Location: On the midline, 3 cun below the umbilicus.
Indications: Urogenital disorders, dysmenorrhea, amenorrhea, cystitis, enuresis. Important for moxibustion in deficiency conditions.
Traditional application: Tonifies the Yin in the body very effectively and nourishes the blood. By tonifying the Yin it also strengthens the Yang Qi, especially kidney Yang.
Needling method: Perpendicular, 2–3 cm.

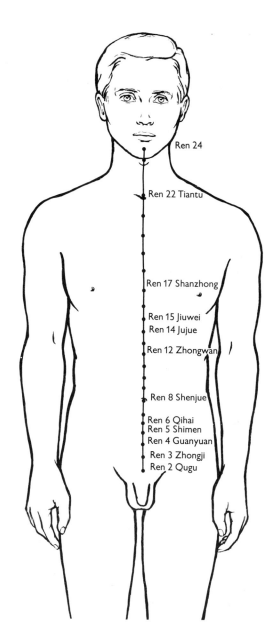

Ren 24

Ren 22 Tiantu

Ren 17 Shanzhong

Ren 15 Jiuwei
Ren 14 Jujue

Ren 12 Zhongwan

Ren 8 Shenjue

Ren 6 Qihai
Ren 5 Shimen
Ren 4 Guanyuan

Ren 3 Zhongji
Ren 2 Qugu

Ren 6 Qihai   Sea of vital energy

Location: On the midline, 1.5 cun below the umbilicus.
Indications: States of weakness. This is a general tonification point and is indicated together with St.36 Zusanli and Sp.6 Sanyinjiao in chronic fatigue, depression, convalescence, and hypotension. Moxibustion should be used.
Traditional application: Tonifies the Yang Qi in thewhole body, as the sea of Qi.
Needling method: Perpendicular, 2–3 cm.

Ren 8 Shenque   Palace gate of the spirit

Location: Umbilicus.
Indications: This point is a forbidden for acupuncture. Moxibustion is useful in abdominal pain and diarrhea. The umbilicus is an important general tonification point, like Ren 6 Qihai.

Ren 12 Zhongwan   In the middle of the stomach pit   **Influential point for the Fu organs, Mu point of the stomach**

Location: On the midline, midway between the xiphoid process and the umbilicus, 4 cun above the umbilicus.
Indications: Gastric and duodenal ulcer, gastritis, nausea, vomiting, abdominal distention, digestive and liver disorders.
Traditional application: Harmonizes spleen and stomach, clears dampness.
Needling method: Perpendicular, 2–3 cm.

Ren 14 Juque   Large palace gate   **Mu point of the heart**

Location: On the midline, 6 cun above the umbilicus.
Indications: Stomach disorders, heart diseases such as angina pectoris, mental disorders such as insomnia and agitation.
Needling method: Perpendicular, 2–3 cm.

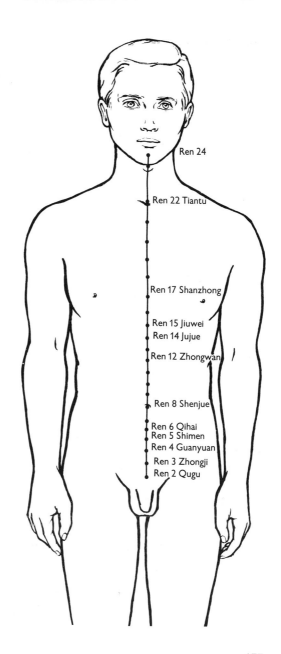

Ren 24

Ren 22 Tiantu

Ren 17 Shanzhong

Ren 15 Jiuwei
Ren 14 Jujue

Ren 12 Zhongwan

Ren 8 Shenjue

Ren 6 Qihai
Ren 5 Shimen
Ren 4 Guanyuan

Ren 3 Zhongji
Ren 2 Qugu

Ren 17 Shanzhong   Middle of the chest   **Mu point of the pericardium, influential point for the respiratory system**

Location: In the middle of the sternum between the nipples, at the level of the 4th intercostal space.
Indications: Heart and lung disorders, bronchial asthma, disorders of the chest wall.
Traditional application: Tonifies Qi, especially in the upper Jiao, i. e. lung and heart. Clears phlegm.
Needling method: Oblique, in a downward direction, 2–3 cm.

Ren 22 Tiantu   Standing out from heaven

Location: In the jugular fossa.
Indications: Acute attacks of bronchial asthma, hiccough, dysphagia, pharyngitis.
Needling method: First the needle is inserted 0.5 cun in a backward direction, after which the patient is asked to lean his or her head right back, and the needle can then be advanced parallel to the posterior border of the sternum 3–4 cm in the caudal direction. This point should be used only by the experienced acupuncturist. Incorrect insertion endangers the great vessels and other vital organs in the mediastinum.

Ren 23 Lianquan   Modest spring

Location: Midway between the upper border of the cricoid cartilage and the lower border of the mandible.
Indications: Aphasia, mutism, dysphagia, speech disorders following stroke, stuttering, hypersalivation, pharyngitis, laryngitis.
Needling method: Oblique toward the root of the tongue, 2–3 cm.

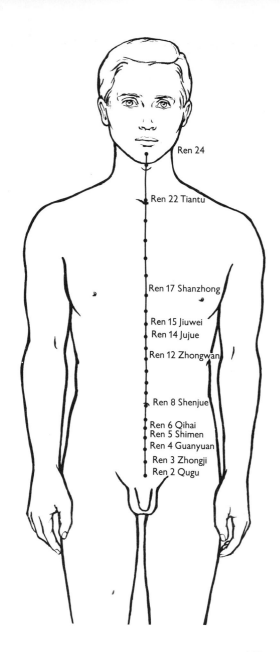

Ren 24

Ren 22 Tiantu

Ren 17 Shanzhong

Ren 15 Jiuwei
Ren 14 Jujue

Ren 12 Zhongwan

Ren 8 Shenjue

Ren 6 Qihai
Ren 5 Shimen
Ren 4 Guanyuan

Ren 3 Zhongji
Ren 2 Qugu

4.4.15 Extra Points Ex.

After the categorization of the 361 classic acupuncture points located on the 14 channels, new points were found and introduced as extra points. In this book the terminology of the Academy of Traditional Chinese Medicine is used. Every point has a Chinese name, which shows its location or function, e.g., Ex.2 Taiyang = temple, Ex.8 Anmian I = silent sleep. Most of the extra points are not located on any of the 14 channels. The acupuncture literature published in recent years differs widely in the numbering systems used for the extra points. In 1984 the World Health Organization established an international standard for acupuncture point names, including the 31 commonly used extra points. The extra points were not numbered by the committee. The use of their Chinese names is particularly important. In this book we also give the numbering system published by the Academy of Traditional Chinese Medicine in 1975 in the book *Outlines*, because it is widely used.

The regions in which the extra points are found are abbreviated by the WHO standardization committee as follows:

Extra points on the head and neck	– Ex-HN
Extra points on the chest and abdomen	– Ex-CA
Extra points on the back of the trunk	– Ex-B
Extra points on the upper extremities	– Ex-UE
Extra points on the lower extremities	– Ex-LE

Only the most important extra points are described.

Extra points on the head and neck   Ex-HN

Ex.1 Yintang   Stamp hall   Ex-HN

Location: Between the eyebrows on the midline at the root of the nose.
Indications: Rhinitis, frontal headache, frontal sinusitis, eye disorders.
Needling method: Oblique, in caudal direction, 0.5 cm.

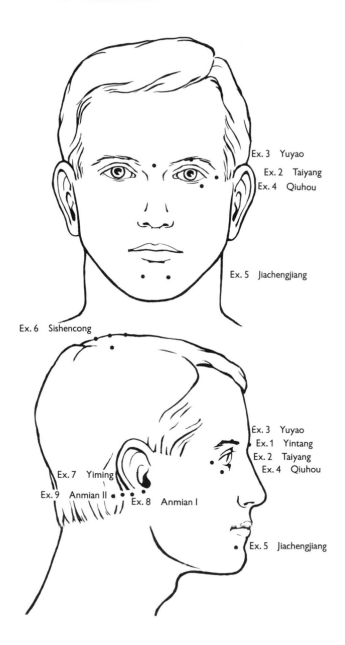

Ex. 3   Yuyao
Ex. 2   Taiyang
Ex. 4   Qiuhou

Ex. 5   Jiachengjiang

Ex. 6   Sishencong

Ex. 3   Yuyao
Ex. 1   Yintang
Ex. 2   Taiyang
Ex. 4   Qiuhou

Ex. 7   Yiming

Ex. 9   Anmian II
Ex. 8   Anmian I

Ex. 5   Jiachengjiang

Ex. 2 Taiyang Temple **Ex-HN**

Location: At the point of intersection of the continuations of the eyebrow and the lower eyelid in the lateral direction, on the lateral border of the orbita.
Indications: Headache, migraine, eye disorders, facial paralysis, trigeminal neuralgia, frontal sinusitis, toothache.
Needling method: Perpendicular or oblique, 1 cm.
A dangerous point.

Ex. 3 Yuyao Fish back **Ex-HN**

Location: In the middle of the eyebrow, directly above the pupil.
Indications: Frontal sinusitis, eye disorders, headache.
Needling method: Oblique, 0.5 cm, in medial direction for frontal sinusitis, in ventral direction for eye disorders.

Ex. 6 Sishencong The four spiritual wise men **Ex-HN**

Location: Four points, located 1 cun anterior, posterior, and lateral to Du 20 Baihui.
Indications: Headache, apoplexy, epilepsy, agitation, insomnia.
Needling method: Oblique, 0.5 cm toward Du 20.
These four points are usually needled together with Du 20.

Ex. 8 Anmian I Calm sleep

Location: Between SJ. 17 Yifeng and Ex. 7 Yiming, 0.5 cun dorsal to SJ. 17.
Indication: Insomnia.
Needling method: Perpendicular, 1 cm. Anmian I and II are used together.

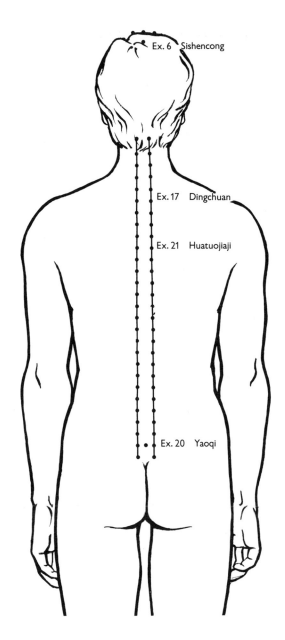

Ex. 6 Sishencong

Ex. 17 Dingchuan

Ex. 21 Huatuojiaji

Ex. 20 Yaoqi

Ex. 9 Anmian II   Calm sleep

Location: Midway between Ex. 7 Yiming and GB. 20 Fengchi.
Indication: Insomnia.
Needling method: Perpendicular, 1 cm.

Extra points on the back   Ex-B

Ex. 17 Dingchuan   Calming asthma

Location: 0.5 cun lateral to Du 14 Dazhui.
Indication: Important point for bronchial asthma.
Needling method: In slightly medial direction, 1 cm.

Ex. 21 Huatuojiaji   Huatuo points bind the spine

This point is named for the famous Chinese surgeon Hua Tuo;
Huatuo means wonderful son.

Location: This is a series of 28 point pairs, located 0.5 cun lateral to
the lower border of the processus spinosus, between C1 and S4.
Indications: Pain along the spine, segmental pain radiation, disorders
of the internal organs corresponding to the segmental innervation.
Needling method: 1 cm in the cervical and thoracic region. The needles should be inserted in a slightly medial direction. Three to five
Huatuo points are used in one acupuncture treatment session.

Extra points on the upper extremity   Ex-UE

Ex. 28 Baxie   Eight obliquities   **Ex-UE**

Location: On the back of the hand, at the midpoints of the webs
(8 points). The patient should form a fist for needling at these points.
Indications: Disorders and pain in the fingers, rheumatoid arthritis.
Needling method: Oblique, in proximal direction, 1 cm.

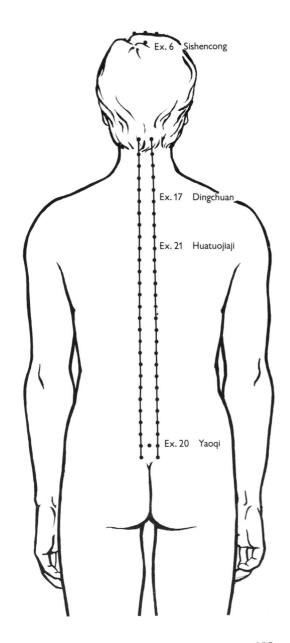

Ex. 6 Sishencong

Ex. 17 Dingchuan

Ex. 21 Huatuojiaji

Ex. 20 Yaoqi

185

Extra points on the lower extremities   Ex-LE

Ex. 31 Heding   Crane crest   **Ex-LE**

Location: At the middle of the upper border of the patella.
Indications: Disorders of the knee joint.
Needling method: Perpendicular, 0.5–2 cm.

Ex. 32 Xiyan   Knee gap   **Ex-LE**

Location: At the level of the lower border of the patella, medial to the ligamentum patellae.
Indication: Disorders of the knee joint.
Needling method: Perpendicular or oblique, in medial direction, 0.5–2 cm. The point St. 35 Dubi, located on the lateral side of the lower border of the patella, is also called lateral Xiyan. These points together with Ex. 31 are indicated as local points for the treatment of disorders of the knee joint.

Ex. 36 Bafeng   Eight winds   **Ex-LE**

Location: On the dorsum of the foot in the middle of the webs, 8 points.
Indications: Arthritis of the toes, pain and paresthesia of foot and toes.
Needling method: Oblique in proximal direction, 1 cm. Liv. 2 Xing-jian, St. 44 Neiting and GB. 43 Xiaxi coincide in location with the Bafeng points.

Neima   (Nei means medial and Ma, anesthesia)

Location: On the posterior border of the tibia midway between the medial malleolus and the knee joint. This point corresponds to the location of Liv. 6 Zhongdu.
Indications: Analgesic point for surgery in the lower abdominal and urogenital areas. This point is indicated for pain relief during childbirth, together with Sp. 6 Sanyinjiao.
Needling method: Perpendicular, 1–2 cm.

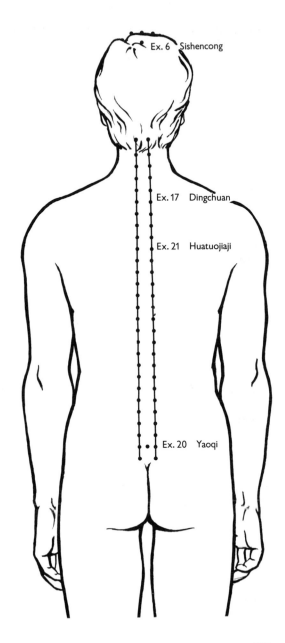

Ex. 6 Sishencong

Ex. 17 Dingchuan

Ex. 21 Huatuojiaji

Ex. 20 Yaoqi

187

5 Technique of Acupuncture

G. STUX

5.1 Acupuncture Needles

Today, mostly filiform steel needles are used for acupuncture. The steel used is flexible and unbreakable. Gold and silver needles are applied very rarely and only in ear acupuncture. The diameter of the needles varies from 0.2 to 0.5 mm and is given often as the gauge (26–32):

Gauge	34	32	30	28	26
mm	0.22	0.26	0.32	0.38	0.45

In most cases needles 0.3–0.4 mm thick are used. The length varies from 1 to 10 cm and is often given in inches, the 1-in., $1^{1}/_{2}$-in., and 2-in. needles being most common. Filiform needles consist of a tip, a body, and a handle. The length of the needles refers to the body. Often the wire webbing handle is made of silver. Double-webbed needles are better for easy manual stimulation and are called dragonhead needles.

During acupuncture the patient should be lying comfortably in the supine position. This is the best position for relaxation of the patient during acupuncture treatment and also the best way of preventing fainting. The patient should not move during treatment, because it can be painful if the needles bend in the muscle. For treatment of points on the back, e.g., in lower back pain, patients should lie prone or in a lateral position. This position should also be comfortable for the patient. Fainting occurs in 5% – 10% of patients treated in the sitting position, especially at the beginning of the treatment.

Acupuncture needles are held vertically between the thumb on one side and the index and middle fingers on the other. The middle finger guides the needle and prevents its bending during insertion. The needles are mostly held perpendicular to the fingers, seldom parallel. The tip of the needle extends 1–5 cm from the point

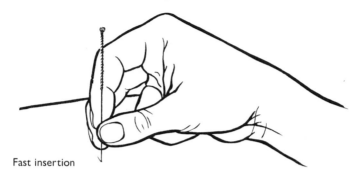

Fast insertion

of contact with the fingers, especially with long needles, which are more liable to bend. Insertion of the needle, especially the perforation of the skin, should be fast. Fast insertion clearly reduces the pain. In the *slow method of insertion* the skin is penetrated slowly during rotation of the needle. The skin can be pressed simultaneously with the nail of the thumb of the free hand. The slow method may be painful, and therefore the fast method is preferred by most Chinese practitioners.

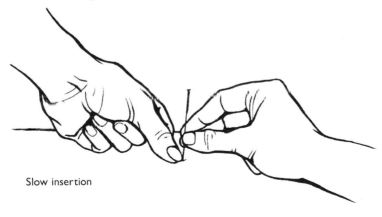

Slow insertion

Beginners can practise the different methods of insertion on a cork, or by needling layers of paper fixed in a frame. When the fast method is tried, the number of layers of paper in the frame should be increased to enhance the resistance. Points should be marked on the paper so that precise insertion of needles can be practised.

During insertion of the needle attention should be focused on its tip. The Chinese say that Qi should be focused into the needle.

The insertion can be perpendicular (90°), or oblique (30°–60°), or occasionally tangential (10°). The depth of insertion and the direction are given with the specific acupuncture point, but they are approximate values, which can vary depending on the constitution of the patient. In children the depth of insertion is significantly less than in adults, in keeping with their size. In the chapter describing the acupuncture points the depth of insertion is given in centimeters or millimeters and not in cun, because the metric values can be remembered better and are easier to judge. The depth of insertion varies between some millimeters and 5 cm or more. After insertion the acupuncture needles are retained in place for 10–30 min. They must not lead to any pain. The patient should not move during this time, because this might cause pain.

5.2 De Qi Sensation

When the needles are inserted and retained in place, patients feel a typical sensation called De Qi by the Chinese. This sensation is subjective and is described as numbness, pressure sensation, heaviness, soreness, or distention. A feeling of heat or of coldness can also be present.

The De Qi sensation differs from patient to patient and is also dependent on the place of needling. It is more pronounced when the point is located in peripheral muscles or when distal points of the hand or feet are needled. It is associated with the feeling of insertion, which is generally felt in deep layers of the tissue.

Often the De Qi sensation radiates along the channel, especially when distal points are needled. Often the patients feel a flowing sensation along the channel or in a particular region of the body.

This phenomenon is called **"propagated sensation along the channel"** (PSC). In recent years much research work has been done in China on this phenomenon, which generally occurs in 5%–10% of patients. Different methods of stimulation of needles can evoke propagated sensations along the channels, which have a positive effect on the success of the treatment. The patients should be encouraged to focus their attention to this feeling of flow and observe it during the treatment session (see Chap. 9).

5.3 Tonifying and Sedating Methods of Stimulation

Manipulation of the needles is essential for classic acupuncture treatment. There are three major techniques for this:

- Lifting and thrusting
- Rotation, clockwise and counterclockwise, at an amplitude of 90°–180°
- Combination of rotation with lifting and thrusting

The effect of acupuncture treatment depends essentially on the stimulation of the needles and whether a clear De Qi sensation was experienced by the patient. If the patient finds it painful, manual stimulation should be discontinued. Therefore, the patient is asked to say whether pain is experienced during manual stimulation.

According to traditional theories there are three major methods of stimulation:

1. **Tonifying method,** Chinese *Bu,* also called strengthening; this is applied in deficiency-type disturbances (Yin type or *Xu* in Chinese) The tonifying method is characterized by careful, pain-free needling with thin needles inserted in the direction of flow in the channel, gentle manipulation or none at all, and long retention of the needles (15–30 min). Quick insertion and slow withdrawal of the needle is also tonifying. *Gentle manipulation* of the needles is the essential factor. Moxibustion, the heating of acupuncture points, is another major method of tonifying.

2. **Sedating method,** in Chinese *Xie,* also called the draining, dispersing, or reducing method; this is applied in excess-type conditions (Yang type or *Shi* in Chinese). For the sedating method the needles are manipulated vigorously following insertion. The needling is performed against the direction of flow in the channel. The retention period is short (10–15 min). Slow insertion followed by quick withdrawal is sedating. Generally, thicker needles are used for sedation than for tonification. *Intensive manipulation* of the needles is essential for the sedating method.

3. The **even method** of needling is technically midway between the tonifying and sedating methods. The spectrum ranges from markedly sedating to intensely tonifying methods.

Table 5.1. Sedating and tonifying methods

Sedation, Xie	Tonifying, Bu
Reducing, dispersing method	Reinforcing, strengthening method
Vigorous, intensive manipulation	Weak stimulation
Thick needles (0.3–0.6 mm)	Thin needles (0.1–0.3 mm)
Brief retention (5–15 min)	Protracted retention (15–30 min)
Against the channel flow	With the channel flow
Counterclockwise	Clockwise
Slow insertion	Quick insertion
Quick withdrawal	Slow withdrawal
Insertion during inhalation	Insertion during exhalation
"Son" sedating point	"Mother" tonifying point
	Moxibustion

5.4 Sterilization of the Needles

Acupuncture needles are generally sterilized with a hot air sterilizer at 180 °C or in an autoclave. Especially because of the danger of contamination with hepatitis or HIV, needles must be sterilized with the utmost care, and the exact time and temperature during sterilization should be carefully controlled.

Disinfection or boiling of needles is totally inadequate. In the recent past years disposable needles have been introduced.

5.5 Complications of Acupuncture Treatment

Acupuncture is a safe method with no side effects when general precautions are observed. Nonetheless, complications can occur, as documented in the literature:

1. **Fainting** during acupuncture treatment occurs mainly in nervous, tense, or tired patients. When acupuncture is performed with the patients in a sitting position, fainting, the most common complication, is seen in about 5%–10%. To avoid this, patients should be treated while lying down.

2. **Local infections** are a very rare complication, because the subcutaneous tissues have a high resistance against the thin acupuncture needle. Local infections are caused by inadequate sterilization or by overtraumatization of the tissue when acupuncture is carried out by an inexperienced therapist. In over 10000 personal cases no abscesses or other evidence of local infections have been seen. In ear acupuncture, however especially when permanent needles are used, local infections of the auricle are reported more often.

3. **Pain** during insertion of the needles is due to clumsy insertion technique or to blunt or hooked needles. If a patient moves during acupuncture treatment this can cause pain, and therefore patients should lie in a stable position and should have the opportunity of communicating any discomfort during the period of needle retention. Tense or anxious patients feel more pain. Needling at points on the face and at Jing points is more painful than elsewhere.

4. **Injuries** to internal organs have been reported in the literature, but such complications are very rare and are caused by insufficient anatomical knowledge. In particular, injury to the lung could be caused by deep needling of points on the chest wall, and therefore the dangerous points in this region should be needled obliquely and to a depth of no more than 1 cm.

5.6 Moxibustion

Zhen Jiu, the Chinese name for acupuncture, meaning needling and burning, also embraces the application of moxibustion. In moxibustion acupuncture points are heated by burning dried leaves of *Artemisia vulgaris.* A. vulgaris is a medicinal herb that is common in both Asia and Europe. The leaves are dried and prepared to give a similar consistency to that of cotton wool.

Often acupuncture and moxibustion are practised together as complementary forms of treatment in the same session. The indications for moxibustion include a wide range of weakness (*Xu*) diseases; it is especially effective in weakness after reconvalescence and in depression:

Chronic bronchitis
Bronchial asthma
Chronic diarrhea
Depression
Bowel disease
Hypotension
Exhaustion
Feeling of coldness in the body
Chronic disease

Moxibustion is contraindicated in fever, in acute infectious diseases, in the presence of hypertension, hemorrhage, and during menstruation, and also in nervousness with sleep disturbances, that is to say in Yang conditions.

Selection of points for moxibustion depends on the individual symptoms of the disease. The principles used in selection of points for moxibustion are similar to those followed for acupuncture, but some special points are favored:

- General tonification points
- Shu and Mu points of the related organs
- Specific tonification points ("mother points") and Yuan points
- The navel, a forbidden point for acupuncture, is an important tonification point for moxibustion

Moxibustion is not applied on the head, in the face, or near to mucous membranes. There are many methods of applying moxibustion:

Indirect Moxibustion with Ginger Slice Isolation

In this method of moxibustion fresh ginger slices 1–2 mm thick are used to isolate the direct heat of the burning moxa leaves. Fresh ginger roots are cut into slices 1–2 cm in diameter and placed on the skin at specific acupuncture points. A cone of moxa wool is put on top of each ginger slice and then ignited. The heat penetrates slowly to the deep layers of the skin. When the patient feels a sensation of heat at one point, the ginger slice with the moxa cone is moved away and placed on the next point, subsequently being returned to the first. In this way every point is heated six to eight times, until a slight redness is observed.

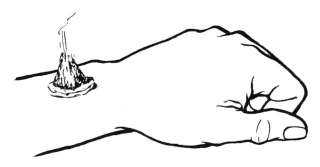

Moxibustion with Ginger slice isolation

This method is very effective, but it should be applied with care so as not to burn the skin, especially when the ginger slice with the burning moxa cone is moved to the next point.

This method can be applied by the patient at home. The practicionar marks the chosen acupuncture points with a permanent felt pen. Then the method is explained in detail to the patient. This can be also done with the help of a video film produced at our center.

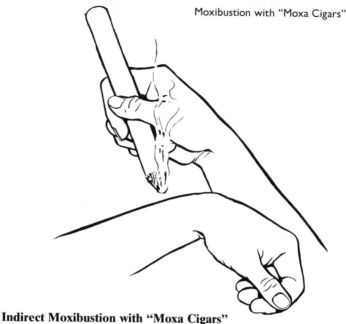

Indirect Moxibustion with "Moxa Cigars"

For this method moxa wands are rolled in thin paper; these are called moxa cigars or moxa rolls. A moxa cigar is ignited in a similar way to an ordinary cigar, at one end, and brought up to only 0.5–1 cm away from the chosen acupuncture point until the patient feels a sensation of heat. The moxa cigar is then removed (3–4 cm) and is brought nearer again after a few seconds. This is repeated six to eight times until a slight redness is observed. In this way, every acupuncture point is heated for about 30–40 s. Care must be taken not to burn the skin. This method has been in wide use since the time of the Ming Dynasty (1368–1644).

Moxibustion by Heating Acupuncture Needles

A small ball of moxa is fixed on the free end of an acupuncture needle and ignited. The heat is conducted through the needle to the deeper layers of the subcutis and muscle. This method is used especially for the Back Shu points and GB.30 Huantiao.

Moxibustion
by heating acupuncture needles

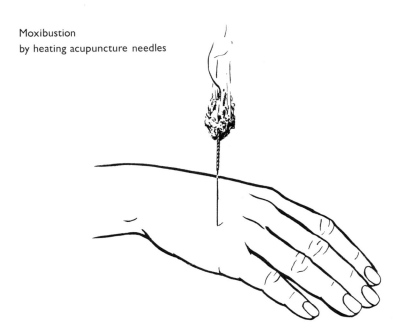

Infrared Moxibustion

Most instruments on the market use infrared radiation directly or
indirectly on the skin. In general the traditional methods seem to
be more effective than infrared moxibustion. However, some patients do not like the smell of burning moxa leaves, and in this
case it is advisable to use infrared moxibustion.

5.7 Acupressure

Acupressure is the massage of acupuncture points. It is indicated in
mild disturbances and diseases. Since ancient times acupressure has
been used as a method of self-care by patients. The major indications
for acupressure are painful conditions such as headache, toothache,
cervical spondylitis, and shoulder and lumbar pain. Many psychosomatic disturbances can also be positively influenced by acupressure,
e.g., sleep disturbances, nervousness, nausea, feeling that vomiting
is imminent, seasickness, constipation, or menstrual problems.

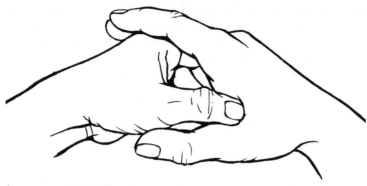
Acupressure of LI. 4 Hegu for pain relief

In acute painful conditions light massage with the pads of the index finger or the thumb is advisable. In chronic diseases moderately vigorous massage is applied. The finger should remain at the same point whether massage is performed with a circular motion or to and fro along the channel. In the case of massage to and fro the pressure in the direction of the channel flow is pronounced. Massage along the channel in its direction of flow is especially effective when the pain is felt along the channel. The pressure exerted by the finger should be light when points over nerves, around sensory organs, or on the frontal side of the neck are massaged and at the beginning of the treatment. The length of time that acupressure should applied is 30–60 s at local points and 1–2 min at distal points. Acupressure can also be used to complement a course of acupuncture treatment in the free interval. As in any form of self-treatment by a patient, before it is attempted a clear Western diagnosis should be made.

5.8 Laser Acupuncture

At the end of the 1960s Mester, in Hungary, began to use low-intensity laser light to treat wounds that were not healing. Probably in 1973, laser light of low intensity was first applied to acupuncture points by Ploog. When these trials were first started laser light with a wavelength of 632 nm in the red visible range, produced by helium neon lasers, was used. A therapeutic effect similar to that of classic acupuncture was observed in some, especially chronic, disorders. This method of irradiating acupuncture points with laser light of low intensity was introduced into the everyday practice of acupuncture in Western Europe at the end of the 1970s.

In 1975 the first *helium neon laser* device with a wavelength of **632 nm** was introduced in Germany. Later *infrared lasers with* **904 nm** wavelength and 10–150 mW intensity generated from gallium arsenide diodes were also manufactured. The latest development are diode laser devices with **780 nm** wavelength and 10–150 mW intensity. These low-energy laser systems are also called **soft lasers.**

The main indications for laser acupuncture are skin diseases and chronic pain conditions, but Ménière's syndrome and mental disorders are also treated by this technique. Especially in children and in oversensitive patients, laser acupuncture has clear advantages. On the other hand, clinical experience shows that in acute painful conditions laser acupuncture has a inferior effect to classic acupuncture. In skin diseases, in addition to the irradiation of acupuncture points, the skin lesions themselves are irradiated, generally for 2 min per cm^2, with lasers of 2 mW intensity. Cosmeticians have also recently started to use this method of irradiating the affected skin area to enhance skin regeneration and improve wrinkles.

In clinical use of laser acupuncture the points are selected in the same way as for classic acupuncture, with 10–20 points irradiated for 10–30 s each per treatment session. Two to three sessions of laser acupuncture are administered per week. Laser irradiation can also be applied to the common points of the ear. Special care must be taken, when laser treatment is applied to points near the eye, **not to radiate directly into the pupil.** Serious harm can be caused to the retina, because the lens of the eye concentrates the laser light many thousand times and it is then focused on the retina. This can also happen with the invisible infrared lasers (780 or 904 nm), if the laser is directed into the pupil. Therefore, the handle should be brought close to the skin before the laser light is turned on. **The patient's eyes should be closed when laser treatment is applied.**

6 Acupuncture Treatment

G. STUX

According to the traditional Chinese view, the cause of an illness lies in a disturbance of the vital energy Qi of organs and channels, that is, in a disharmony of Yin and Yang of the life forces. Therefore, the primary aim of the treatment is to balance Yin and Yang, thus harmonizing the flow of Qi. Much attention is devoted to the prophylaxis of illnesses. A harmonious way of life that strengthens the body and its resistance (*Wei Qi*) is recommended. This includes balanced nutrition, regular physical and breathing exercises (e.g., *Qi Gong,* later *Tai Ji Quan*), and psychic harmony in social life. A long life in harmony with the surrounding nature and society was aspired to.

When illnesses occurred, first the life forces were strengthened. Then the disturbances of the channels and organs concerned were systematically combated by eliminating pathogenic influences to harmonize the excess or deficiency conditions. Apart from acupuncture and moxibustion, herbs were used in treatment.

According to Chinese medicine no separation of psyche and soma was known. The human being was considered in its wholeness, in association with the rest of nature and the social milieu.

In the first part of this chapter the principles of acupuncture and the rules of point selection are presented, in the second part the specific acupuncture treatment of the main disorders.

6.1 Principles of Acupuncture and Rules of Point Selection

Important bases for a successful acupuncture treatment are:

- Comprehensive **diagnosis with the methods of Western medicine,** with particular emphasis on the exclusion of malignant illnesses.
- Exact **analysis of the symptoms** and, especially in chronic and complicated cases, classification of them **according to the system of traditional diagnosis.** The differentiation with the most bearing on therapy is that into excess or deficiency conditions. Disturbances caused by excess, *Shi* in Chinese, are treated with sedative methods, while deficiency disturbances, *Xu,* are treated with tonifying methods. Moxibustion is an important tonifying method. Points should be selected with careful reference to these diagnostic categories, especially in organic disorders.
- Examination and **allocation of pain and of other symptoms to channels and organs.**
- Knowledge of the 12 main channels, and of Ren Mai and Du Mai, their courses, their relations, and the distribution of specific points. Knowledge of the point categories, their indications and meanings.
- **Exact location of the points, precisely correct technique of insertion,** an adequate depth of needle insertion, and appropriate stimulation (sedative or tonifying method).

In point selection for treatment, major empirical principles and rules based on the traditional knowledge of Chinese medicine are used. They have been extended through the findings of modern scientific research over the past 30 years.

1. Every acupuncture point has a **local effect** on the surrounding area.
2. Painful, indurated (e. g., myogelosis), and tender points are also used as local acupuncture points. They are called **locus dolendi points,** in Chinese **Ah Shi points.**
   The **trigger points** in trigeminal neuralgia should not be needled in acute conditions, because this can increase the pain.

3. Every acupuncture point has an effect on disturbances of the **corresponding channel,** coupled channel and on illnesses of the corresponding organ and allocated tissues and sensory organs (Table 6.1).
   These principles of acupuncture are basic to point selection.
4. Acupuncture points have an effect on the related **channel axis,** for example St. 38 Tiaokou along the Yang-Ming (stomach-large intestine). This is an important rule for the treatment of exterior conditions like locomotor disorders.
5. Points located distal to the elbow and knee are called **distal points** and have an influence on proximal areas. The distal

Table 6.1. Interelation of organ, tissue, sensory organ, and element

Zang organs	Fu organs	Tissue	Sensory organs	Phases
Lung	Large intestine	Skin, body hair	Nose	Metal
Kidney	Bladder	Bone, joints	Ear	Water
Liver	Gallbladder	Muscle, tendon	Eye	Wood
Heart	Small intestine	Blood, blood vessels	Tongue	Fire
Pericardium	Sanjiao			
Spleen	Stomach	Connective tissue, "flesh"	Mouth	Earth

Table 6.2. Six important distal points

	Point	Location	Proximal area
Arm	**LI. 4 Hegu**	Between thumb and index finger	Face, neck, sensory organs
	Lu. 7 Lieque	1.5 cun proximal to the wrist joint on the radial border	Neck, lung
	Pe. 6 Neiguan	On the inner side of the forearm, 2 cun proximal to wrist joint	Epigastrium The front of chest
Leg	**St. 36 Zusanli**	Lateral to the shin bone below the knee	Organs of the abdomen
	UB. 40 Weizhong	In the middle of the popliteal crease	Low back, urogenital organs
	Sp. 6 Sanyinjiao	3 cun above the medial malleolus	Pelvic organs, perineum

points listed in Table 6.2 are chosen frequently. Apart from their distal effects on the head, neck, face, and epigastrium, they have important general effects, e.g., analgesia.

Apart from these six distal points, numerous points located distal to the elbow and knee have a specific effect on proximal regions.

6. Some distal acupuncture points have pronounced **analgesic, sedative, immune-enhancing, tonifying, or homeostatic effects** (Table 6.3).

7. For symptomatic treatment acupuncture points with **specific effects** are used (Table 6.4).

8. The **five Shu points** distal to the elbow and knee correspond to the five phases and are used in treatment according to traditional Chinese rules. The five Shu points Jing, Ying, Shu/Yuan, Jing and He are also applied individually. They have different effects and indications:

Jing points (Wade-Giles: *Ting*) are the most distally situated points and are located at the corners of fingernails and

Table 6.3. Specific points

Points with analgesic effect	LI.4	Hegu
	St.44	Neiting
	St.43	Xiangu
Points with tonifying effect	Ren 6	Qihai
	Ren 8	Shenque
	St.36	Zusanli
	Sp.6	Sanyinjiao
Points with sedative effect	Du 20	Baihui
	Ex.6	Sishencong
	He.7	Shenmen
	UB.62	Shenmai
Points with homeostatic effect	LI.11	Quchi
	Sp.6	Sanyinjiao
	St.36	Zusanli
Points with immune-enhancing effect	LI.11	Quchi
	Du 14	Dazhui
	Du 13	Taodao

Table 6.4. Symptomatic points

Symptom	Points
Hiccough	St. 36, Pe. 6, UB. 17
Nausea	Pe. 6, St. 36
Sweating	He. 6, Ki. 7, LI. 4
Sneezing	LI. 20, Ex. 1, Pe. 6
Edema	Sp. 9, Ren 5, Ren 9
Insomnia	Du 20, He. 7, Ex. 8, Ex. 9
Fever	Du 14, LI. 11, LI. 4
Constipation	SJ. 6, St. 25
Diarrhea	Sp. 4, St. 36, Ren 6

toenails. They are selected in acute emergencies (e. g., collapse, shock, nausea). According to Chinese thinking, in extreme deficiency conditions, for example collapse, the Yang energy returns to the channel when Jing points are needled. The point Du 26 Renzhong, located below the nose, is the most important Jing point. Needling of Jing points is mostly painful. In acute emergencies, if no needle is on hand, the Jing points should be pressed with the fingernail.

9. At the **Yuan point,** the Luo connection which comes from the Luo point of the coupled channel ends. According to the traditional view, most of the organ energy along the channel course is concentrated at this Yuan point. The Luo and Yuan points are chosen in disturbances of the coupled Zang and Fu organs. Many important and frequently used acupuncture points are Yuan points; for example LI. 4 Hegu is the most important analgesic point, He. 7 Shenmen one of the most effective harmonizing points.

10. **He points** are the most proximally situated Shu points and are found in the area of the elbow or knee. According to Chinese medicine, at this point the river of Qi flows from the periphery into the sea of the body organs. The He points are important in the treatment of illnesses caused by external factors. Many of the frequently used acupuncture points are He points, e.g., LI. 11 Quchi, St. 36 Zusanli, Sp. 9 Yinlingquan, UB. 40 Weizhong, GB. 34 Yanglingquan, and Liv. 8 Ququan.

11. According to traditional rules, the five Shu points include a **tonification point** and a sedative point. The tonification point corresponds to the "mother element" according to the law of the five phases and tonifies the Qi of the corresponding channel and organ. The tonification points are selected in deficiency conditions of organs and channels. Moxibustion is often applied.

12. The **sedative point**, the "son element" according to the law of the five phases, is also one of the five Shu points. The Qi of channels and organs is sedated at this point. The sedative points are needled in excess conditions and are stimulated with sedative methods.

13. The **Luo point** is the starting point for the Luo vessel that connects this point with the Yuan point of the coupled channel, e.g., Lu.7 Lieque (Luo) with LI.4 Hegu (Yuan). The Luo point is also connected to the corresponding internal organ and has a strong effect on it. The Luo points are frequently selected for treatment of the internal Zang and Fu organs, for example Lu.7 Lieque in lung, St.40 Fenglong in stomach, and He.5 Tongli and Pe.6 Neiguan in cardiovascular disorders.

14. **Xi-cleft points** (Wade-Giles: *Trsi*) are chosen in acute conditions of the corresponding internal organs (e.g., acute gastritis, acute bronchitis). According to traditional ideas the Xi-cleft points activates the flow of energy in the channels and thus of the organs. They are vigorously stimulated.

15. Apart from their other effects, the **eight influential points** have a specific influence on the tissues and organ systems and the functions corresponding to them (Table 6.5).

Table 6.5. Influential points

Tissues, organs	Influential points	
Zang organs, storage organs	Liv.13	Zhangmen
Fu organs, hollow organs	Ren 12	Zhongwan
Respiratory system	Ren 17	Shanzhong
Blood	UB.17	Geshu
Bone	UB.11	Dashu
Bone marrow	GB.39	Xuanzhong
Muscle, tendon	GB.34	Yanglingquan
Vascular system	Lu.9	Taiyuan

16. **Mu points or alarm points** (Wade-Giles: *Mo*) are sensitive to pain and vary in consistency in acute and chronic disturbances of the corresponding organs. They are important in diagnosis as well as in treatment. The Mu points are situated ventrally on the trunk (Table 6.6). They have a similar function to the Back Shu points.

17. The **Back Shu points or transport points** (Wade-Giles: *Yu*) are located segmentally on the medial branch of the urinary bladder channel. Like the alarm points, the Back Shu points become sensitive to pressure in disturbances of the corresponding organ. Apart from their diagnostic relevance, the Shu points are important for the treatment of organ disorders. According to traditional ideas the Shu points transport directly the vital energy, Qi, to the related internal organs. The Shu points are often used together with the Mu points in treatment of illnesses of the internal organs, particularly in chronic conditions (Table 6.7). In deficiency conditions of the organs, moxibustion of the Shu and Mu points is very effective.

18. **Points are selected with reference to the innervation** of the dermatome or myotome or to the corresponding peripheral nerves in neuralgia and neurological disorders. The **Huatuojiaji points (Ex. 21)** situated 0.5 cun lateral to the vertebral column in each

Table 6.6. Mu or alarm points

Organs	Mu points	
Lung	Lu. 1	Zhongfu
Pericardium	Ren 17	Shanzhong
Heart	Ren 14	Juque
Liver	Liv. 14	Qimen
Gallbladder	GB. 24	Riyue
Spleen	Liv. 13	Zhangmen
Stomach	Ren 12	Zhongwan
Sanjiao	Ren 5	Shimen
Kidney	GB. 25	Jingmen
Large intestine	St. 25	Tianshu
Small intestine	Ren 4	Guanyuan
Urinary bladder	Ren 3	Zhongji

Table 6.7. Back Shu points

Organs	Back Shu points		Location
Lung	UB.13	Feishu	T3
Pericardium	UB.14	Jueyinshu	T4
Heart	UB.15	Xinshu	T5
Liver	UB.18	Ganshu	T9
Gallbladder	UB.19	Danshu	T10
Spleen	UB.20	Pishu	T11
Stomach	UB.21	Weishu	T12
Sanjiao	UB.22	Sanjiaoshu	L1
Kidney	UB.23	Shenshu	L2
Large intestine	UB.25	Dachangshu	L4
Small intestine	UB.27	Xiaochangshu	S1
Urinary bladder	UB.28	Pangguangshu	S2

segment and the points on both branches of the urinary bladder channel are especially effective.

19. **Unilateral disorders** can also be treated with points on both sides of the body. This is effective and should be borne in mind during selection of the distal points that are regularly needled on both sides. In *acute* trigeminal neuralgia only local points on the contralateral side are used at the beginning of treatment, while distal points on both sides are stimulated.

Many principles of acupuncture treatment are based on traditional ideas of pathology and diagnosis. This book describes only the important rules of point selection.

The next part of this chapter deals with the point combinations that are used in important disorders and have been confirmed in daily practice. In 1979 the World Health Organization drew up an indication list of the important disorders for which acupuncture treatment (Appendix A). The spectrum of acupuncture indications treated in this book goes beyond the WHO list and includes most disorders that are treated with acupuncture in Western countries.

The point combinations listed below should not be uncritically followed like recipes but should help the beginner to get a "feel" for point selection.

An analysis of the point combinations with reference to the principles of acupuncture presented is especially instructive. The selection of points for a particular disorder must take account of the **individual symptoms.** The detail following system of treatment is based on Western diagnosis. Study of the traditional syndromes of Chinese medicine is recommended for the advanced acupuncturist.

A **holistic concept** of acupuncture should be maintained. The combination of dietary advice, physical therapy, and psychotherapy can be of decisive importance in healing. Drug treatment, if indicated, should be slowly reduced.

Du 20 Baihui, the "governor" of the Du Mai, the governing vessel, is the point that effects central coordination of all Yang points. In addition, Du 20 is an effective sedative and harmonizing point. Therefore, this point can be used in every acupuncture treatment.

Generally two treatment sessions are carried out per week. In acutely painful conditions, such as trigeminal neuralgia, acute migraine, or pain in carcinoma, daily treatment can be useful. An interruption of 7–14 days is inserted after 8–12 sessions.

In general the needles are retained in place for 10–25 min and then removed; but retention for up to 1 h can be necessary in trigeminal neuralgia or pain in carcinoma.

In all displayed lists of indications below, the acupuncture points are listed in this way: 1st column, local points; 2nd column, distal points on the arms; and 3rd column, distal points on the legs. The important points are always listed first.

According to the individual symptoms, 10–15 of the listed points are selected, so that a **maximum of 20 needles per acupuncture treatment** are used. These points can be varied individually.

Before every acupuncture treatment, points that are painful or sensitive to pressure in the diseased region, the so-called Ah Shi points, are searched for and used as local acupuncture points.

6.2 Locomotor Disorders

The effect of acupuncture treatment in these disorders has been verified by many controlled studies. The good results of acupuncture treatment in such chronic pain conditions are verified in daily practice.

Principles of treatment:

- Points that are painful and sensitive to pressure, **Ah Shi points,** are systematically selected and needled.
- The location of **pain and its radiation must be related to the channels** to allow treatment by needling of specific local and distal points of the appropriate channel. For example, pain in the shoulder along the large intestine channel is treated with local points on the large intestine channel and with important distal points, such as LI.4 Hegu, LI.11 Quchi.
- In pain along a channel, points of the **corresponding axis** are also selected; for example, in pain along the large intestine channel, points of the stomach channel, of the Yang-Ming (e.g., St.38 Tiaokou), are used.
- The **influential point for muscles and tendons, GB.34 Yanglingquan,** is indicated in all disorders of muscles and tendons.
- In degenerative disorders of joints, bone, and cartilage the **influential point UB.11 Dashu** is selected.
- **Analgesic points,** such as **LI.4 Hegu and St.44 Neiting,** are often additionally used in pain treatment.

6.2.1 Cervical Spondylitis, Torticollis, Rheumatoid Arthritis

According to Chinese classification cervical spondylitis is differentiated into two forms according to pain location:

- In the first type the pain occurs **near the midline,** indicating that it is related to the small intestine channel. Pain is characterized by restricted movements and by an increase when tilting the head forward or backward. Corresponding local points and dis-

tal points on the small intestine and urinary bladder channels are
selected for treatment.
– When there is pain along the **lateral side** of the neck and restricted movements and pain on turning the head, cervical spondylitis
is treated with the Sanjiao and gallbladder channels.

In acute cervical spondylitis and torticollis, stimulation with a sedative method is necessary, that is, vigorous manipulation of the
needle. In chronic cases moxibustion is indicated in addition to
tonifying needling.

Cervical spondylitis medial Tai Yang type
(small intestine and urinary bladder channels)

Du 20 Baihui		
UB.10 Tianzhu	SI.3 Houxi	UB.60 Kunlun
Du 14 Dazhui	SI.6 Yanglao	
UB.11 Dashu	Lu.7 Lieque	
Ex.21 Huatuojiaji	LI.4 Hegu	
Ah Shi points		

Cervical spondylitis lateral Shao Yang type
(Sanjiao and gallbladder channel)

Du 20 Baihui		
GB.20 Fengchi	SJ.5 Waiguan	GB.39 Xuanzhong
GB.21 Jianjing	LI.4 Hegu	GB.34 Yanglingquan
Du 14 Dazhui		
Ah Shi points		

6.2.2 Intercostal Neuralgia,
Trauma of the Thorax, Ankylosing Spondylitis,
Zoster Neuralgia

In severe cases acupuncture treatment should be administered over
20–30 sessions. In such long-term cases with typical deficiency
symptoms, moxibustion is indicated in addition. Even in chronic
and severe zoster neuralgia high degrees of success are achieved.

Du 20 Baihui
Ex.21 Huatuojiaji   SJ.8 Sanyangluo   GB.40 Qiuxu
Segmental urinary   LI.4 Hegu
bladder points UB.11–UB.21 (3–5 points)
Ah Shi points

6.2.3 Sciatica, Lumbar Pain

Sciatic pain is related either to the urinary bladder channel (medial) or to the gallbladder channel (lateral). Differentiation into acute types with Yang character or chronic types with deficiency symptoms is indispensable for treatment to be effective. In the cases of acute onset of disease and severe pain, vigorous manipulation of the acupuncture needles is applied. Electrical stimulation can be helpful. In chronic cases with dull pain, deficiency symptoms, and sensitivity to cold, in addition to needling, moxibustion is indicated. According to Chinese ideas there is a deficiency of the kidney Yang in such cases. Moxibustion of the corresponding specific points (UB.23, UB.25, Ki.7, Ki.8, Sp.6) is then applied (see Chap.8).

Pain along the urinary bladder channel – Tai Yang Type

Du 20 Baihui
Du 3   Yaoyangguan   LI.4 Hegu   UB.40 Weizhong
Du 4   Mingmen   Hand point 1   UB.60 Kunlun
UB.23 Shenshu   UB.58 Feiyang
UB.25 Dachangshu   UB.57 Chengshan
UB.26 Guanyuanshu
UB.54 Zhibian
UB.36 Chengfu
Ah Shi points

Pain along the gallbladder channel – Shao Yang Type

Du 20 Baihui
GB.30 Huantiao   LI.4 Hegu   GB.34 Yanglingquan
GB.31 Fengshi   GB.39 Xuanzhong
Du 3   Yaoyangguan
Du 4   Mingmen

Points for moxibustion

UB.23 Shenshu	Ki.7 Fuliu
UB.25 Dachangshu	Ki.3 Taixi
Du 3 Yaoyangguan	Sp.6 Sanyinjiao

UB.26–30 Paravertebral line connecting sacral urinary bladder points

6.2.4 Periarthritis Humeroscapularis, Frozen Shoulder

Local points in the area of the shoulder girdle are selected according to the location of the most pain:

- In pain located on the anterior side of the shoulder, points on the large intestine channel (LI.15, 16) on the shoulder are needled together with distal points of this channel (LI.4, 11) and with the important distal point at the leg (St.38) of the Yang-Ming (large intestine and stomach).
- If pain is located on the dorsal side of the shoulder joint, local points on the small intestine channel (SI.9–11) are used in combination with distal points of this channel (SI.6).
- In the case of pain in the middle of the shoulder, local and distal points of the Sanjiao channel are selected. An additional point of reference in selection of the appropriate channel is yielded by differentiation of the symptoms into restricted and painful movements of the shoulder joint:

Anteversion – **large intestine channel (Yang-Ming)**
Abduction – **Sanjiao channel (Shao-Yang)**
Retroversion – **small intestine channel (Tai-Yang)**

In painful restricted movements of the shoulder joint (frozen shoulder), stimulation of **St.38 Tiaokou** is very effective. In a personal study 40% of the patients had recovered after the first session and 80% after two or three treatments.

Pain on the frontal side of the shoulder (Yang-Ming)

Du 20 Baihui
LI.15 Jianyu   LI.4   Hegu   St.38 Tiaokou
LI.16 Jugu   LI.11 Quchi
LI.14 Binao

Pain in the middle of the shoulder (Shao-Yang)

Du 20 Baihui
SJ.14 Jianliao   SJ.5   Waiguan
SJ.13 Naohui   LI.4   Hegu   St.38 Tiaokou

Pain on the dorsal side of the shoulder (Tai-Yang)

Du 20 Baihui
SI.9   Jianzhen   SI.6   Yanglao
Du 14 Dazhui   SI.3   Houxi

6.2.5 Epicondylitis, Tennis Elbow

In treatment of the very painful condition of epicondylitis, great
care must be devoted to the selection of points that are painful or
tender on pressure. Distal points of the corresponding channel are
added. Vigorous stimulation, especially of the distal points, is very
effective. Sudden movements of the joint and heavy carrying must
be avoided.

Du 20 Baihui
LI.11 Quchi   LI.4   Hegu
Lu.5   Chize   SJ.5   Waiguan
Pe.3   Quze
He.3   Shaohai
Ah Shi points are very important.

6.2.6 Coxarthrosis, Coxarthritis

According to traditional ideas coxarthrosis is mostly caused by a deficiency-type disturbance. Treatment with a tonifying method is indicated. Especially in predominantly dull and numbing pain, needling and moxibustion of the tonification points is successful.

Du 20 Baihui		
GB.30 Huantiao	LI.4 Hegu	GB.34 Yanglingquan
UB.54 Zhibian		UB.40 Weizhong
UB.32 Ciliao		UB.60 Kunlun
UB.36 Chengfu		St.44 Neiting
Ah Shi points		

Points for moxibustion

UB.23 Shenshu	UB.40 Weizhong
UB.54 Zhibian	Ki.3 Taixi
	Ki.7 Fuliu

6.2.7 Gonarthrosis, Pain in the Knee Joint

The three local points, Ex.31 Heding, Ex.32 Xiyan, and St.35 Dubi, which are also called knee eyes, are central to the treatment, and painful local points and points tender to pressure are also selected. Distal points on the appropriate channels related to the local points are vigorously stimulated.

Du 20 Baihui		
Ex.31 Heding	LI.4 Hegu	St.44 Neiting
Ex.32 Xiyan	UB.11 Dashu	UB.60 Kunlun
St.35 Dubi		
St.36 Zusanli		
GB.34 Yanglingquan		
UB.40 Weizhong		
Ah Shi points		

Swelling of the joints

Sp.9 Yinlingquan

6.2.8 Rheumatoid Arthritis

According to Chinese medicine there is a traditional syndrome, called *Bi,* that is similar in its symptoms to rheumatoid arthritis. The **Bi syndrome** is caused by a disturbance of the Qi and blood flow. Pathogenic influences such as wind, cold, damp, and a deficiency of the protecting Qi (Wei-Qi) provoke this disease. Several forms of the Bi syndrome are differentiated:

1. Bi syndrome with severe pain that is relieved by heat. The cause is *pathogenic cold.*
2. Bi syndrome with vagrant pain sensations and restricted movements, caused by *pathogenic wind* influence.
3. Bi syndrome with long-lasting pain, heaviness, and physical sluggishness, caused by *pathogenic damp.*
4. Bi syndrome with acutely inflamed joints (swelling, redness, heat), caused by a combination of *pathogenic cold, dampness, and wind.*

The traditional therapy eliminates the pathogenic influences of cold, damp, and wind and enhances the body's resistance. Because primarily a deficiency is involved, the treatment is based on activation of the Qi by means of moxibustion at tonification points. Needling of the appropriate channels and joints eliminates the pathogenic influence. Moxibustion of general and specific tonification points is carried out daily.

Needle treatment in combination with moxibustion is indicated for quite a long period. Antirheumatic drugs should be reduced slowly, in keeping with the pain relief achieved with acupuncture. The following point are general tonification points for needling and moxibustion.

Ren 6	Qihai	LI.11	Quchi	St.36	Zusanli
Ren 8	Shenque	LI.10	Shousanli	Ki.7	Fuliu
Ren 12	Zhongwan	Lu.9	Taiyuan	Sp.6	Sanyinjiao
UB.20	Pishu				
UB.22	Sanjiaoshu				
UB.23	Shenshu				
Du 4	Mingmen				
Du 13	Taodao				
Du 14	Dazhui				

The influential point for muscles and tendons, GB.34 Yangling-quan, is very effective in rheumatic illnesses. UB.11 Dashu, the influential point for bone and cartilage, is often needled. In acute inflammations Du 14 Dazhui is indicated. Long-term treatment often not only reduces the pain but also improves the movement in the affected joints.

6.3 Respiratory Disorders

Many respiratory disorders are successfully treated by acupuncture. Especially in chronic conditions, such as chronic sinusitis, bronchitis, or bronchial asthma, acupuncture is more effective than other forms of treatment. Long-term success can be frequently achieved even in therapy-resistant cases. In acute infections of the upper respiratory system, the acute symptoms can usually be alleviated within a short time (one or two treatment sessions).

According to traditional medicine, external climatic influences such as cold, wind, dryness, and occasionally heat are considered to be causal factors, together with a weakened lung. Excess- or deficiency-type disturbances (Shi and Xu forms) can occur. Their differentiation is important for point selection and for the technique of stimulation.

Principles of treatment:

– **Local points** in the area of the disorder:

Nose: LI. 20 Yingxiang, Ex. 1 Yintang
Maxillary sinus: LI. 20 Yingxiang, St. 2 Sibai, St. 3 Juliao, SI. 18 Quanliao
Frontal sinus: UB. 2 Zanzhu, GB. 14 Yangbai, Ex. 3 Yuyao, Ex. 1 Yintang
Tonsils: Ren 23 Lianquan, LI. 18 Neck Futu, SI. 17 Tianrong

– **Important distal points** for respiratory disorders:

Lu. 7 Lieque	Luo point of the lung with a strong effect on the respiratory system.
LI. 4 Hegu	Specific effect on the head and neck; decreases fever and increases sweating; as Yuan point of the large intestine, it connects with the Luo vessel to the lung channel (Lu. 7). This point eliminates pathogenic influences.
Lu. 6 Kongzui	Xi-cleft point of the lung, indicated in acute cases of bronchitis or asthma.

SJ.5 Waiguan Eliminates the heat-type symptoms and other climatic influences, similar to LI.4.

- **Ren 17 Shanzhong, the influential point** for the respiratory system, is selected especially in bronchitis and asthma.

- **The Shu and Mu points** of the lung, **UB.13 Feishu** and **Lu.1 Zhongfu,** are selected in deficiency disturbances (Xu) of the lung and are stimulated with tonifying method. In this case moxibustion of these points is also indicated.

- **Ex.17 Dingchuan** is a specific extra point for relief of asthma.

- **Ren 22 Tiantu** is effective in **acute attacks of asthma.**

- **UB.17 Geshu** has a relaxing effect on the diaphragm and stimulation of this point is indicated in cough and dyspnea caused by asthma.

- **St.40 Fenglong** increases expectoration of persistent and viscous mucus.

- Local points in the area of the disorder with a specific effect on disturbances caused by wind (Feng), such as GB.20 Fengchi, Du 16 Fengfu, UB.12 Fengmen for the common cold.

- **Du 14 Dazhui,** LI.11 Quchi, and LI.4 Hegu are effective in relief of fever.

- **He.7 Shenmen** and **Pe.6 Neiguan** are useful if **psychogenic factors** are predominant.

6.3.1 Common Cold

According to traditional ideas, common cold is caused by external pathogenic climatic factors such as cold and wind, occasionally heat, in association with weakened lung Qi and weakened defense (Wei Qi). The typical symptoms, such as headache, pains in the limbs, exhaustion, and tiredness, are an expression of the external factors. Symptoms like fever, thirst, and dryness of the mucous membranes are present in heat-type disturbances, when the fluid (Yin) is exhausted.

Du 20 Baihui		
GB.20 Fengchi	Lu.7 Lieque	Sp.10 Xuehai
Du 14 Dazhui	LI.4 Hegu	St.44 Neiting
Du 16 Fengfu	LI.11 Quchi	Liv.3 Taichong
	SJ.5 Waiguan	

The treatment is aimed at expelling the external pathogenic factors and especially at activating the protective forces of the lung.

In the second phase of the disorder, when the acute symptoms have been attenuated, moxibustion of the points listed below is advisable. Moxibustion can be carried out daily by the patient.

LI.11   Quchi
Ren 6   Qihai
St.36   Zusanli
Ki.7   Fuliu
UB.12   Fengmen

6.3.2 Maxillary Sinusitis

Acupuncture is especially effective in a chronic course of this disease. The relapse rate can be significantly reduced.

Du 20 Baihui		
LI.20 Yingxiang	LI.4 Hegu	Sp.10 Xuehai
St.2 Sibai	LI.11 Quchi	St.44 Neiting
St.3 Juliao		
SI.18 Quanliao		

6.3.3 Frontal Sinusitis

In frontal sinusitis such symptoms as frontal headache and a sensation of pressure between the eyes are effectively relieved.

Du 20 Baihui		
UB.2 Zanzhu	LI.4 Hegu	UB.60 Kunlun
Ex.3 Yuyao	LI.11 Quchi	St.44 Neiting
Ex.1 Yintang		
GB.14 Yangbai		

6.3.4 Chronic Bronchitis

According to traditional ideas a deficiency-type disturbance of the lung is accompanied often by a deficiency of the kidney or spleen. The treatment is based on activation of the organ systems and on a harmonizing influence on the lung function.

Du 20 Baihui		
Lu. 1 Zhongfu	Lu. 9 Taiyuan	St. 40 Fenglong
UB. 13 Feishu	Lu. 7 Lieque	St. 36 Zusanli
Du 14 Dazhui		
Ren 17 Shanzhong		

UB. 17 Geshu has a calming effect in chronic cough.

If deficiency symptoms caused by a chronic course are predominant, moxibustion is useful.

UB. 13 Feishu	Lu. 9 Taiyuan
UB. 20 Pishu	LI. 11 Quchi
UB. 23 Shenshu	
Du 4 Mingmen	
Ren 6 Qihai	

According to traditional ideas acute bronchitis is caused by an external wind or cold influence, and it is therefore considered an excess-type disturbance. The treatment is similar to that for the common cold.

6.3.5 Bronchial Asthma

In acute forms long-lasting success can be achieved. Even after a course over some decades with chronic effects on the lung, bronchospasm can be reduced.

Asthma is divided into excess and deficiency types (Shi and Xu forms). Asthma of the excess type is caused by external wind and cold influences or by heat, in which case it is characterized by stagnation and accumulation of sputum. In asthma of the deficiency type, the kidney is also often in a deficiency state. The differentiation of excess and deficiency types according to traditional diagnostic categories is essential for treatment.

Asthma of excess type

Du 20   Baihui
Ren 17 Shanzhong   Lu.7 Lieque   St.40 Fenglong (in
UB.13 Feishu   LI.4 Hegu   case of blocked mucus)
Lu.1   Zhongfu   Lu.5 Chize (in heat-type disturbance)
Ex.17 Dingchuan   Lu.6 Kongzui (in acute shortness of breath)
Ren 22 Tiantu (in acute shortness of breath)   Ki.3 Taixi
Du 14   Dazhui (in acute infection)

Asthma of deficiency type

Du 20   Baihui
Ren 17 Shanzhong   Lu.9 Taiyuan
UB.13 Feishu   Lu.7 Lieque
Ex.17 Dingchuan

In asthma of deficiency type, in addition to needling with tonifying stimulation (mild stimulation), moxibustion is very important. Moxibustion of the following tonification points is applied daily:

UB.13 Feishu   Lu.9 Taiyuan   St.36 Zusanli
UB.23 Shenshu   LI.11 Quchi   Ki.3   Taixi
Du 4   Mingmen
Ren 6   Qihai
UB.20 Pishu in deficiency of the spleen together with
Ren 12 Zhongwan

6.4 Cardiovascular Disorders

An exact Western diagnosis must be made before acupuncture treatment. Other possible therapies should be used in addition to acupuncture if indicated. In cardiovascular disorders acupuncture is used very effectively. Acupuncture is especially appropriate for the treatment of psychosomatic heart disorders. In hypotension, hypertension, and exhaustion conditions resulting from chronic heart disorders, a combination of acupuncture and moxibustion is effective.

6.4.1 Coronary Heart Disease with Angina Pectoris

In coronary heart disease acupuncture should be carried out in association with drug treatment. Acupuncture has a sedative and harmonizing effect on the heart. According to traditional ideas stagnation of Qi and blood of the heart is present.

Du 20	Baihui		
UB.15	Xinshu	Pe.6	Neiguan
Ren 14	Juque	He.7	Shenmen
Ren 17	Shanzhong	Pe.4	Ximen (in acute conditions)

6.4.2 Cardiac Neurosis

In cardiac neurosis the psychogenic character is predominant. The patients suffer from anxiety, restlesness, internal agitation, nervousness, palpitation, and tachycardia and have pains in the chest and along the inner side of the left arm (heart channel). According to the concepts of traditional medicine an excess-type disturbance is present in such cases. After a few acupuncture sessions the physical symptoms are significantly reduced, and the patient's anxiety and nervousness are attenuated.

Du 20	Baihui		
Ex.6	Sishencong	He.7	Shenmen
Ren 14	Juque	He.5	Tongli
Pe.1	Tianchi	Pe.6	Neiguan

6.4.3 Exhaustion Conditions in Heart Disease

According to traditional ideas a deficiency of the heart and of other organ systems, e.g., the kidney or spleen, is often diagnosed. In these deficiencies moxibustion of important Shu and Mu points has a tonifying effect. General tonification points are also helpful in such cases. Needling of important points of the heart and pericardium channels has a harmonizing effect.

Points for moxibustion

UB.15	Xinshu
UB.20	Pishu
UB.21	Weishu
UB.23	Shenshu
Ren 6	Qihai
St.36	Zusanli
Ren 14	Juque
Ren 12	Zhongwan
GB.25	Jingmen

Points for acupuncture

Du 20	Baihui		
Ren 17	Shanzhong	He.7	Shenmen
Ren 14	Juque	Pe.6	Neiguan

6.4.4 Hypertension

According to traditional ideas an excess-type disturbance of the liver with a deficiency of the kidney is present in hypertension. Needling and stimulation of Liv.3 Taichong, the Yuan point of the liver, balances this disturbance very effectively; since it causes a pronounced reduction in blood pressure patients should be treated only in a lying position. Vigorous stimulation enhances the effect of the antihypertensive treatment. During acupuncture treatment medication should be reduced according to the blood pressure.

Du 20	Baihui				
Ex.6	Sishencong				
UB.15	Xinshu	LI.11	Quchi	Liv.3	Taichong
GB.20	Fengchi	He.7	Shenshu	St.36	Zusanli
				Liv.2	Xingjian

6.4.5 Hypotension

In hypotension many typical deficiency symptoms are present: dizziness, tiredness, feeling of weakness, shivering, cold feet and hands. The treatment is mostly based on moxibustion of important tonification points.

UB.23 Shenshu	LI.11 Quchi	St.36 Zusanli
Ren 6 Qihai	LI.10 Shousanli	Ki.7 Fuliu
Du 12 Shenzhu		
Du 11 Shendao		

Besides moxibustion, needling of these points with a tonifying method is also indicated.

6.4.6 Disturbances of Peripheral Blood Supply

According to traditional ideas a stagnation of Qi and blood is present. Acupuncture treatment re-establishes the disturbed flow of Qi and blood. Important homeostatic points, such as LI.11 Quchi and St.36 Zusanli, together with the influential point for blood vessels, Lu.9 Taiyuan, and Ex.28 and Ex.36, Baxie and Bafeng, are effective. Vigorous manual stimulation is necessary. Moxibustion can be useful, but burnings must be avoided, made more likely by reduced sensitivity of the skin.

Du 20 Baihui		
UB.15 Xinshu	Lu.9 Taiyuan	GB.34 Yanglingquan
Ren 17 Shanzhong	LI.11 Quchi	St.36 Zusanli
	He.3 Shaohai	Ex.36 Bafeng
	Ex.28 Baxie	Liv.3 Taichong
	LI.4 Hegu	

6.5 Gastroenterological Disorders

Especially in functional and psychosomatic gastroenterological disorders, acupuncture treatment is very successful. The traditional diagnostic categories of excess and deficiency must be differentiated. Excess-type disturbances, e.g., gastritis or ulcers, are treated with vigorous needle manipulation (sedative), while in deficiency-type disturbances moxibustion is indicated.

The following points are very effective in the treatment of gastrointestinal disorders:

- **St. 36 Zusanli** is the most important distal point for gastrointestinal disorders. Personal studies have verified the spasmolytic effect of this point by gastroscopic monitoring.

- **Pe. 6 Neiguan** has a specific effect on the upper digestive tract and is effective in nausea, hiccough, and vomiting.

- **Alarm points** are often used
Ren 12	Zhongwan	for stomach
St. 25	Tianshu	for large intestine
Ren 4	Guanyuan	for small intestine
Liv. 6	Zhongdu	for liver
Ex. 35	Dannang	for gallbladder
Ex. 33	Lanwei	for appendix

- **Shu points** are useful in chronic disorders
UB. 21	Weishu	for stomach
UB. 20	Pishu	for spleen
UB. 22	Sanjiaoshu	for Sanjiao
UB. 18	Ganshu	for liver
UB. 19	Danshu	for gallbladder

Moxibustion is applied to the Shu and Mu points for the corresponding functional systems.

6.5.1 Gastritis, Gastroenteritis

In acute gastritis, according to traditional criteria such excess-type symptoms as heartburn, feeling of fullness, and acute pain in the epigastrium are predominant. In gastroenteritis intestinal symptoms often occur in addition. Sedative acupuncture treatment harmonizes the stomach and digestive organs within a short time.

In chronic gastritis a deficiency-type disturbance with symptoms such as loss of appetite, general tiredness, and a sensation of emptiness in the stomach area are present. In addition to needling (tonification method) moxibustion is also indicated, especially at Shu and Mu points on the stomach and spleen channels.

Du 20	Baihui		
Ren 12	Zhongwan	Pe.6 Neiguan	St.36 Zusanli
St.21	Liangmen	He.7 Shenmen	St.34 Liangqiu
St.25	Tianshu		
UB.21	Weishu		
Liv.13	Zhangmen		

Points for moxibustion in chronic deficiency-type disturbances of the digestive tract:

Shu points	**Mu points**	
UB.21 Weishu	Ren 12 Zhongwan	St.36 Zusanli
UB.20 Pishu	Liv.13 Zhangmen	

6.5.2 Gastric and Duodenal Ulcers

As in gastritis, differentiation of excess-type from deficiency-type symptoms according to traditional criteria must precede treatment with a sedative or a tonifying method.

If there is acute and cramp-type pain in the hypochondriac area, a disturbance of the liver may be present; treatment should be at points Liv. 14 Qimen and Liv.3 Taichong, to harmonize the Qi of the liver.

Acute ulcer pain is generally attenuated after some hours. Acute pain is treated daily, and two treatment sessions per week are then given until the ulcer is healed.

Du 20	Baihui				
St. 21	Liangmen	Pe. 6	Neiguan	St. 36	Zusanli
St. 25	Tianshu	He. 7	Shenmen	Sp. 4	Gongsun
Ren 12	Zhongwan			St. 44	Neiting
UB. 21	Weishu			Liv. 3	Taichong
UB. 20	Pishu				
Sp. 15	Daheng				
Liv. 14	Qimen				
Ren 6	Qihai				

6.5.3 Diarrhea

The treatment of diarrhea has a long tradition in China. Diarrhea can also reflect either an excess-type or a deficiency-type disturbance. In acute gastroenteritis the diarrhea is of an excess type with a feeling of fullness and acute, sometimes cramping pain. Vigorous manipulation of the needles, i. e., sedative treatment, brings about fast improvement.

In chronic diarrhea a deficiency-type disturbance of the spleen, and occasionally of the kidney, is present. Moxibustion and tonifying treatment are indicated.

Du 20	Baihui				
St. 25	Tianshu	Pe. 6	Neiguan	Sp. 4	Gongsun
UB. 25	Dachangshu	LI. 11	Quchi	St. 37	Shangjuxu
St. 29	Guilai	LI. 4	Hegu	St. 36	Zusanli
Ren 6	Qihai			Sp. 6	Sanyinjiao
Ren 4	Guanyuan			St. 39	Xiajuxu

Moxibustion in diarrhea with deficiency-type symptoms

St. 25	Tianshu	LI. 11	Quchi	Sp. 4	Gongsun
UB. 20	Pishu			Sp. 6	Sanyinjiao
Liv. 13	Zhangmen			St. 36	Zusanli

Ren 6   Qihai
Ren 4   Guanyuan
UB. 23   Shenshu (in kidney Yang deficiency)
Du 4   Mingmen

6.5.4 Irritable Bowel Disease

The symptoms vary and are characterized by various combinations of constipation and/or diarrhea, abdominal pain, sometimes mucus in the stool, flatulence, and vegetative symptoms. Mental stress is very significant in the etiology of this psychosomatic disorder.

As in other disorders of the digestive organs, the symptoms are differentiated according to traditional diagnostic categories: excess-type disturbances with damp-heat in the large intestine are apparent in acute cramping pain, acute diarrhea, or spastic constipation. Deficiency-type disturbances are characterized by chronic constipation or chronic diarrhea with weakness symptoms, such as dull pain, lack of appetite, tiredness, depressive mood or anxiety state. Moxibustion is advisable in such cases, while in disturbances of the excess type, vigorous needling is indicated.

It is mostly the large intestine that is affected, and therefore St. 37 Shangjuxu, the lower He point of the large intestine, and St. 25 Tianshu, the Mu point of the large intestine, are very important.

Du 20	Baihui				
St. 25	Tianshu	LI. 4	Hegu	St. 37	Shangjuxu
St. 29	Guilai	LI. 11	Quchi	St. 36	Zusanli
Sp. 15	Daheng	Pe. 6	Neiguan	Sp. 4	Gongsun
UB. 25	Dachangshu				
UB. 20	Pishu				
Liv. 13	Zhangmen				

In deficiency-type disturbances moxibustion of Mu and Shu points of the large intestine, spleen, and sometimes stomach channels is indicated.

6.5.5 Constipation

As in irritable bowel disease, the points are selected according to the individual symptoms. The large intestine channel is important for treatment. SJ.6 Zhigou is a very effective point in chronic constipation.

Du 20	Baihui				
St.25	Tianshu	SJ.6	Zhigou	St.37	Shangjuxu
Sp.15	Daheng	LI.11	Quchi	St.36	Zusanli
St.29	Guilai	LI.4	Hegu	Sp.4	Gongsun
UB.25	Dachangshu				

In chronic, deficiency-type disturbances moxibustion is indispensable in addition.

6.5.6 Cholangitis, Cholecystitis, Biliary Dyskinesia, Biliary Colic

Disorders of the biliary ducts are effectively treated with acupuncture, which is indicated especially in chronic and functional disorders. An excess-type disturbance of the liver and gallbladder is usually present. In treatment important points on these channels are used together with the appropriate Shu and Mu points.

Du 20	Baihui				
GB.24	Riyue	LI.4	Hegu	GB.34	Yanglingquan
Liv.14	Qimen	Pe.6	Neiguan	GB.37	Guangming
UB.19	Danshu			Sp.6	Sanyinjiao
UB.18	Ganshu			Liv.3	Taichong
St.21	Liangmen			Ex.35	Dannang
GB.21	Jianjing			St.36	Zusanli
				Liv.6	Zhongdu

6.6 Mental Disturbances and Illnesses

In Western Europe and America acupuncture treatment is increasingly being applied in mental illnesses. Together with psychotherapy, acupuncture, with its various psychic and somatic effects, replaces medication.

Acupuncture has a mental harmonizing, sedative, or tonifying effect. Points of the Du Mai, heart, pericardium, and gallbladder channels have psychological effects.

In many mental disturbances additional organ systems are affected. These organs are treated by stimulation of the points of the corresponding channels. The following points are selected frequently:

Du 20	**Baihui**	the governing point of the Du Mai
Ex. 6	**Sishencong**	with pronounced psychological effect
He. 7	**Shenmen**	Yuan and sedative point of the heart channel
Pe. 6	**Neiguan**	Luo point of the pericardium channel
UB. 62	**Shenmai**	with harmonizing effect
UB. 15	**Xinshu**	the Shu point of the heart channel

Acupuncture treatment is very effective in a large number of psychosomatic disorders, such as agitation or exhaustion conditions, insomnia, depression, sexual disturbances, drug addictions, obesity, and headache; this has been documented by many clinical trials.

6.6.1 Depression

In Chinese medicine depressive disorders are described as a deficiency (Xie) of the kidney Yang. The Chinese understanding of the kidney is mainly based on its function and includes the function of the urogenital system in general, but also the function of the adrenal gland. The function of the will is the psychological correlate. Deficiency of the kidney Yang means a weakened ego.

The symptoms of a kidney Yang deficiency are characterized by pallor, excessive feeling of cold, cold feet and hands, tiredness, reduced activity, lack of energy, and depressed mood. In the case of more severe deficiency disturbances, somatic symptoms are predominant, such as pronounced feelings of cold in the lumbar region, rigidity of the lower back, lumbar pain and sciatica, and reduced libido or impotence. Diminished vitality, lack of drive, and withdrawal from the environment are additional mental symptoms.

Moxibustion is the major treatment method, and the indirect methods with moxa cigars or with moxa cones on slices of ginger are preferred. Moxibustion can be carried out by the patients following demonstration of the method by the doctor. This gives the patients the feeling that they are able to do something for their own health and take responsibility rather than passively having treatment administered by the physician, and this in itself has a positive influence.

The selection of points for moxibustion is dependent on the individual symptoms. The following points have shown their effectiveness in daily practice:

UB. 23	Shenshu	Shu point of the kidney
GB. 25	Jingmen	Mu point of the kidney
Ren 6	Qihai	"sea of vital energy," important general tonification point
Ren 4	Guanyuan	"enclosed source energy," important tonification point
Ren 8	Shenque	navel, important tonification point for moxibustion
Ki. 7	Fuliu	tonification point of the kidney channel
Ki. 8	Jiaoxin	enhances the effect of Ki. 7 Fuliu
Sp. 6	Sanyinjiao	"junction of the three Yin channels," spleen, kidney and liver, important general tonification point
St. 36	Zusanli	general tonification point
Liv. 8	Ququan	tonification point of the liver channel
Lu. 9	Taiyuan	tonification point of the lung channel
LI. 11	Quchi	tonification point of the large intestine channel

Agitated patients with nervousness and restlessness are sedated by stimulation of points on the heart channel. Further harmonizing points of the Du Mai and pericardium channels are added.

Acupuncture of the following points:

Du 20 Baihui
Ex. 6 Sishencong   He. 7 Shenmen   Liv. 3 Taichong
Ren 6 Qihai   He. 5 Tongli   Sp. 6 Sanyinjiao
                    Pe. 6 Neiguan
                    LI. 4 Hegu

6.6.2 Exhaustion Conditions

Typical somatic weakness symptoms such as lack of vitality, tiredness, reduced activity, dizziness, and sensitivity to cold are predominant in this disorder. The weakened organs should be determined. As in depressive illness, the kidney Yang is often weakened. Other organs, i.e., spleen, liver, or lung are also often affected by deficiency states. The basic treatment is moxibustion, which could be combined with acupuncture.

Moxibustion

UB. 23 Shenshu   LI. 11 Quchi   Ki. 7 Fuliu
UB. 22 Sanjiaoshu   SJ. 3 Zhongzhu   Sp. 6 Sanyinjiao
GB. 25 Jingmen   Lu. 9 Taiyuan   St. 36 Zusanli
Ren 6 Qihai
Du 4   Mingmen

Acupuncture

Du 20 Baihui
Du 14 Dazhui   He. 7 Shenmen   St. 36 Zusanli
UB. 15 Xinshu   Pe. 6 Neiguan   Sp. 6 Sanyinjiao
Ren 6 Qihai   Liv. 3 Taichong

6.6.3 Agitation

According to traditional criteria agitation is interpreted as an excess-type disturbance of the heart or of the liver. Acupuncture has a significant sedative and harmonizing effect.

Du 20	Baihui				
Ex. 6	Sishencong	He. 7	Shenmen	Liv. 3	Taichong
UB. 15	Xinshu	Pe. 6	Neiguan	UB. 62	Shenmai
		He. 5	Tongli		

6.6.4 Sleep Disturbances

According to traditional criteria of diagnosis, an excess-type disturbance is present. Deficiency-type conditions, for example of the kidney, can also cause sleep disturbances, especially in old age. The additional symptoms, such as agitation, nervousness, lack of concentration, tiredness, and various vegetative physical symptoms, are related to other disturbed organ systems. They are treated with acupuncture or, in the case of a deficiency, with moxibustion. The major points for sleep disturbance are completed with two specific extra points, Ex. 8 Anmian I and Ex. 9 Anmian II. Anmian in Chinese means "sleep well."

After a few acupuncture sessions the medication taken by most of these patients can be discontinued.

Du 20	Baihui				
Ex. 6	Sishencong	He. 7	Shenmen	UB. 62	Shenmai
Ex. 8	Anmian I	Pe. 6	Neiguan	Sp. 6	Sanyinjiao
Ex. 9	Anmian II			Liv. 3	Taichong
Ex. 1	Yintang				

Moxibustion in deficiency-type disturbances

UB. 23	Shenshu	LI. 11	Quchi	Sp. 6	Sanyinjiao
UB. 22	Sanjiaoshu			Ki. 7	Fuliu
Ren 6	Qihai			Ki. 8	Jiaoxin

6.6.5 Drug Addiction

Acupuncture treatment for patients addicted to opiates was started by the neurosurgeon Wen in Hong Kong in the 1960s. Surprisingly, these patients had no withdrawal symptoms in the acute phase. At first no explanation could be found. Then, in 1979, raised levels of endorphins were demonstrated in heroin addicts treated with acupuncture. Acupuncture treatment in drug addiction, besides discontinuing withdrawal symptoms, and craving for the drugs, also has a psychologically stabilizing effect. Nevertheless, the success of treatment is dependent on the therapeutic circumstances, the attendant psychotherapeutic measures, and the social conditions.

In the 1970s M.O.Smith began treating heroin and cocaine addiction at Lincoln Hospital, Bronx, New York. The results of this treatment were so successful that after a short time 250 patients were coming for daily acupuncture. Many clinical studies show that 60–68% of the patients discontinued taking drugs, determined by urine testing. Smith's drug treatment model has now been introduced into more than 400 treatment facilities all over the world.

Both body acupuncture and specific ear points are used for drug addiction. The points Ear Shenmen, Ear kidney, and Ear heart are very effective.

Smith treats only with ear acupuncture using Ear Shenmen (55), Ear Heart (100), Ear Liver (98), Ear Kidney (95) and Ear Sympathicus (17, Nogier's Nr.22 and 24).

According to traditional Chinese diagnostic criteria a syndrome of "empty fire" i.e., kidney Yin deficiency in combination with Yang excess with excessive fire is predominant in drug-addicted patients.

Du 20 Baihui
Du 14 Dazhui   He.7 Shenmen   St.36   Zusanli
Ear point 55 Shenmen Pe.6 Neiguan   GB.34 Yanglingquan
Ear point 100 heart   LI.4 Hegu   Liv.3   Taichong
Ear point 98 liver   SJ.5 Waiguan
Ear point 95 kidney
Ear point 17 sympathicus (Nogier's 22 and 24)

6.6.6 Alcohol Addiction

Acupuncture treatment of addictions, the therapeutic circumstances and the social conditions are very important for the success of treatment. Mostly the organs stomach-spleen and liver-gallbladder are disturbed. Points on the heart channel have a sedative effect, and the specific ear points relieve the withdrawal symptoms. According to Chinese concepts, a liver Yin deficiency is found here.

Du 20	Baihui		
Ren 12	Zhongwan	He.7 Shenmen	St.36 Zusanli
Liv.13	Zhangmen	Pe.6 Neiguan	GB.34 Yanglingquan
Liv.14	Qimen		Liv.3 Taichong

Ear point 55 Shenmen
Ear point 84 mouth
Ear point 87 stomach
Ear point 98 liver
Ear point 17 sympathicus

6.6.7 Nicotine Addiction

Acupuncture treatment is also very effective in patients who wish to discontinue smoking. The withdrawal symptoms, such as internal agitation, nervousness, excessive appetite, desire for cigarettes, but also sweating, palpitation, and further vegetative physical symptoms, are relieved by acupuncture. As in all drug addictions patient motivation is important for the success of treatment. After patients have discontinued smoking, they are treated two or three times per week, for four or five sessions.

Du 20 Baihui
Ex.6 Sishencong   He.7 Shenmen
Du 14 Dazhui   Pe.6 Neiguan
Ear point 55 Shenmen
Ear point 101 lung
Ear point 87 stomach
Ear point 91 large intestine (in excessive appetite or constipation)
Ear point 17 sympathicus

6.6.8 Overweight, Weight Loss

Acupuncture reduces excessive appetite. According to traditional criteria overweight patients are characterized by deficiency-type disturbances, most frequently of the stomach-spleen system but in some cases even of the kidney. Excessive appetite is an expression of a weakened spleen-stomach system. Therefore, moxibustion is indicated in weight loss in addition to needling.

Treatment of overweight is most effective when accompanied by a course of fasting for 1–2 weeks. During this time the patient should drink 3–4 liters of fluids per day. After fasting the patient can change his or her nutritional habits and adopt a healthy diet much more easily. An individual dietetic consultation is of decisive importance for long-term success of the treatment. Acupuncture treatment should be given two or three times per week, and six to eight times altogether.

Du 20   Baihui
Ren 12 Zhongwan   He. 7 Shenmen   St. 36 Zusanli
Ear point 55 Shenmen Pe. 6 Neiguan   Liv. 3 Taichong
Ear point 87 stomach
Ear point 84 mouth
Ear point 17 sympaticus

Moxibustion in weakness symptoms

Shu points	Mu points	Additional points
UB. 20 Pishu	Liv. 13 Zhangmen	LI. 11 Quchi
UB. 21 Weishu	Ren 12 Zhongwan	St. 36 Zusanli
UB. 23 Shenshu	GB. 25 Jingmen	Ki. 7 Fuliu

6.7 Neurological Disorders

Acupuncture shows a good effect especially in migraine, chronic headache, and trigeminal neuralgia. In these illnesses acupuncture is significantly more beneficial than other therapeutic measures. The sensational successes achieved in these conditions have enhanced the spread of acupuncture in the West. More than 30% of the patients receiving acupuncture in the West suffer from headache or migraine. Even with paralysis acupuncture treatment improves the function of movement, which cannot be achieved with other forms of treatment. In patients with epilepsy acupuncture has a surprising anticonvulsive effect in acute attacks. It is even possible to reduce the relapse rate.

6.7.1 Headache and Migraine

According to traditional ideas chronic headache and migraine are attributed to a blockage of Qi in the Yang channels of the head. The blockages and therefore the pain are mostly caused by an internal disturbance of organs and channels and rarely by external influences caused by weather factors. The location of pain is very important for the planning of an individual acupuncture treatment. According to the traditional concept of Chinese medicine the location and radiation of pain can be divided into four major groups depending on the channels affected:

- **Pain along the gallbladder channel,** with most pain in the area of GB.14 Yangbai above the eyes or GB.20 Fengchi in the neck. Because the pain is localized on the Sanjiao-gallbladder axis, this headache is called **Shao-Yang type headache.** Accounting for 40%–50% of headaches, the Shao-Yang type is the most frequent.

Headache of Shao-Yang type

Du 20 Baihui		
GB.14 Yangbai	SJ.5 Waiguan	GB.41 Foot Linqi
GB.20 Fengchi	LI.4 Hegu	GB.37 Guangming
GB.8 Shuaigu		St.44 Neiting
		Liv.3 Taichong

- **Pain in the area of the temple,** with most pain in the region of St. 8 Touwei, is related to the stomach channel. Such headaches are called **Yang-Ming type headaches** and are treated with distal points of the large intestine and stomach channels.

Headache of Yang-Ming type

Du 20 Baihui		
St. 8 Touwei	LI. 4 Hegu	St. 44 Neiting
GB. 4 Hanyan	LI. 11 Quchi	St. 36 Zusanli

- **Pain along the urinary bladder channel,** with most pain in the area of UB. 2 Zanzhu between the eyebrows or UB. 10 Tianzhu in the neck is called a **Tai-Yang type headache.** Needling and stimulation of distal points on the small intestine and urinary bladder channels is indicated.

Headache of Tai-Yang type

Du 20 Baihui		
UB. 2 Zanzhu	SI. 3 Houxi	UB. 60 Kunlun
UB. 10 Tianshu	LI. 4 Hegu	UB. 67 Zhiyin

- **Pain in the area of vertex Du 20 Baihui** is related to the liver channel. According to traditional ideas an internal connection passes from the liver channel to the point Du 20 Baihui at the vertex. Treatment at distal points of the liver channel is indicated.

Headache in disturbance of liver functions

Du 20 Baihui		
Ex. 6 Sishencong	LI. 4 Hegu	Liv. 3 Taichong
Liv. 14 Qimen	SJ. 6 Waiguan	Liv. 2 Xingjian
		GB. 34 Yanglingquan

6.7.2 Trigeminal Neuralgia

According to traditional ideas trigeminal neuralgia is the result of a blockage of Qi caused by wind, cold, or heat, together with pronounced internal disturbances of the liver or stomach. These organs may be either in an excess state, with heat symptoms and acute burning pain, or in a deficiency state, with dull nagging pain. If periodic or moving pains occur in attacks, a wind disturbance is present. In the treatment of trigeminal neuralgia a large number of points in the face (10–12) are needled on the contralateral side; they should be manually stimulated over and over again, for sedative stimulation. Distal points, especially LI.4 Hegu, are vigorously stimulated by hand.

At first severe cases are treated daily, and the needles are left in for 30–60 min. *In severe acute pain only the contralateral side* of the face should be needled, because the pain might be increased by needling on the painful side. After the acute pain has abated, the painful side can be needled, first of all with a few needles and then gradually increasing their number. The intensity of stimulus given by manual needle manipulation is also slowly increased. In the majority of patients the first alleviation of pain is experienced after four to six sessions. From this time onward drug treatment can be slowly reduced. For a significant pain reduction it is generally necessary to treat for a further 15–20 sessions. After a course of treatment the patients are mostly painfree for several years. When trigeminal pain recurs a new course of treatment with fewer sessions should be administered. According to the location of pain the following points are selected:

Pain in the area of ophthalmicus (V 1)

Du 20	Baihui				
GB.14	Yangbai	LI.4	Hegu	St.44	Neiting
Ex.2	Taiyang	SJ.5	Waiguan	Liv.3	Taichong
UB.2	Zanzhu			St.36	Zusanli
Ex.1	Yintang				

Pain in the area of maxillaris (V 2)

Du 20	Baihui				
St. 2	Sibai	LI. 4	Hegu	St. 44	Neiting
St. 3	Juliao	SJ. 5	Waiguan	Liv. 3	Taichong
SI. 18	Quanliao			St. 36	Zusanli
Du 26	Renzhong				
St. 7	Xiaguan				
LI. 20	Yingxiang				

Pain in the area of mandibularis (V 3)

Du 20	Baihui				
St. 4	Dicang	LI. 4	Hegu	St. 44	Neiting
St. 6	Jiache	SJ. 5	Waiguan	Liv. 3	Taichong
St. 7	Xiaguan			St. 36	Zusanli
Ren 24	Chengjiang				
Ex. 5	Jiachengjiang				

6.7.3 Hemiparesis

The treatment of hemiparesis occupies a major place in acupuncture clinics in China. Hemiparesis after a cerebral insult has a better prognosis than posttraumatic hemiparesis. Paresis after poliomyelitis can also be treated successfully. Personal experience in the treatment of spastic paresis shows a significant reduction of the spasm in 30% of patients. Early treatment of paresis after cerebral palsy has especially good results. Even in long-standing paresis amazing improvements are often achieved.

According to Chinese ideas a pronounced deficiency disturbance is present in paresis, accompanied by a blockage of Qi and blood. Pathogenic internal wind disturbance is also often found. The large intestine and stomach channels are primarily affected, i.e., the Yang-Ming, so that points on them are mostly indicated, with deep needling into the muscles. Electrical stimulation intensifies the effect of acupuncture and counteracts muscular atrophy. Moxibustion is also useful for pronounced cold and weakness symptoms and provides supplementary tonification for the weakened patient.

In the treatment of paresis acupuncture is carried out for two to three cycles of treatment, each of 10–12 sessions. If there is no success of treatment after one cycle, scalp acupuncture should be tried.

Hemiparesis of the arms

Du 20	Baihui				
Ex.6	Sishencong	LI.15	Jianyu	GB.34	Yanglingquan
		LI.11	Quchi		
		LI.10	Shousanli		
		LI.4	Hegu		
		Ex.28	Baxie		
		SJ.14	Jianliao		
		SJ.5	Waiguan		
		SJ.3	Zhongzhu		

Hemiparesis of the legs

Du 20	Baihui	LI.4	Hegu	St.32	Femur Futu
Ex.6	Sishencong	LI.11	Quchi	St.36	Zusanli
St.31	Biguan			St.37	Shangjuxu
				St.40	Fenglong
				St.41	Jiexi
				St.44	Neiting
				Ex.36	Bafeng
				GB.30	Huantiao
				GB.34	Yanglingquan
				GB.37	Guangming
				GB.40	Qiuxu
				Liv.3	Taichong

Points for moxibustion

Ren 6	Qihai	LI.10	Shousanli	St.36	Zusanli
Ren 4	Guanyuan	LI.11	Quchi	Sp.6	Sanyinjiao
UB.23	Shenshu	SJ.5	Waiguan	St.41	Jiexi
UB.25	Dachangshu				

6.7.4 Facial Paresis, Bell's pulsy

Electrical stimulation with low frequencies of 3–10 Hz intensifies the effect of needling. The local points are stimulated only on the affected side, while the distal points are stimulated on both.

Du 20	Baihui					
Ex. 6	Sishencong	LI. 4	Hegu	GB. 34	Yanglingquan
GB. 14	Yangbai	LI. 11	Quchi	St. 36	Zusanli
Ex. 2	Taiyang			St. 44	Neiting
St. 2	Sibai				
St. 3	Juliao				
St. 4	Dicang				
St. 5	Daying				
St. 7	Xiaguan				
SI. 18	Quanliao				
Ex. 5	Jiachengjiang				

6.7.5 Epilepsy

Acupuncture treatment has good anticonvulsive effects, especially in the treatment of acute attacks. Needling or pronounced acupressure with the fingernail leads to interruption of the convulsion within seconds in a high percentage of patients. In acute attacks the point **Du 26 Renzhong** is very effective in 80%–90% of the patients, which is verified by personal research results. In an emergency a thin disposable cannula can also be used.

Long-term treatment is also effective in the interval between epileptic attacks. Medication should first be continued until constant relief from attacks is obtained and then slowly reduced in consultation with the attending neurologist.

Treatment of attacks

Du 26 Renzhong

Treatment in interval between epileptic attacks

Du 20 Baihui

Ex.6 Sishencong	He.7 Shenmen	Ki.1 Yongquan
Ex.1 Yintang	Pe.6 Neiguan	UB.62 Shenmai
Du 26 Renzhong	LI.4 Hegu	GB.34 Yanglingquan
		Liv.3 Taichong

6.8 Gynecological Disorders

According to the concepts of traditional Chinese medicine, the genital organs are related to the kidney system. The liver channel is also important, because it passes along the genital area. The Ren Mai, also called the conceptional vessel, is closely related to the genital organs. Therefore, gynecological disorders are treated with points on the kidney and liver channels, Ren Mai, and Du Mai. The differentiation into excess- or deficiency-type disturbances is very important for the success of treatment, determining whether the emphasis should be on needle treatment or moxibustion. Many disorders are caused by deficiency-type disturbances, of the kidney system for example.

The most important points for urogenital disorders are the same as for urological ones, listed below (see Sect. 6.9).

6.8.1 Dysmenorrhea

According to traditional ideas either an excess-type disturbance with cramp-type pain is present, which increases with pressure or warmth and radiates into the legs or the back, or rarely a deficiency-type disturbance, which is characterized by dull pain during or after menstruation, that is relieved by warmth and pressure. Dizziness, tiredness, or sensitivity to cold may also be present. In excess-type disturbances the blockage of Qi and blood is treated with strong stimulation, i.e., a sedative method. In the deficiency-type disturbance, besides needling, moxibustion of the Mu and Shu points of the kidney is indicated but not during menstrual bleeding.

Du 20	Baihui		
Ren 3	Zhongji	LI. 4 Hegu	Sp. 6 Sanyinjiao
Ren 6	Qihai		Sp. 10 Xuehai
Ren 4	Guanyuan		Liv. 3 Taichong
St. 29	Guilai		St. 36 Zusanli

Moxibustion in deficiency disturbance

UB. 23 Shenshu	GB. 25 Jingmen	Sp. 6 Sanyinjiao
UB. 20 Pishu	Liv. 13 Zhangmen	Ki. 7 Fuliu
Ren 4 Guanyuan		St. 36 Zusanli
Ren 6 Qihai		Ki. 3 Taixi

6.8.2 Pain Caused by Gynecological Tumors

Acupuncture, because of its good analgesic effects, is indicated in tumor pain of the pelvic region. Acupuncture is especially advisable because the general condition is mostly poor and acupuncture has no side effects such as strong analgesic drugs do. In severe pain electrical stimulation with changing impulses is very effective.

According to Chinese concepts in cancer extreme deficiency of Yin, the structural force is present.

Du 20 Baihui		
Ren 4 Guanyuan	LI. 4 Hegu	Sp. 6 Sanyinjiao
Du 3 Yaoyangguan	LI. 11 Quchi	St. 44 Neiting
UB. 23 Shenshu		Liv. 3 Taichong
UB. 25 Dachangshu		

Tonifying with moxibustion in poor general condition

UB. 23 Shenshu	LI. 11 Quchi	Sp. 6 Sanyinjiao
GB. 25 Jingmen		St. 36 Zusanli
UB. 26–30		UB. 40 Weizhong
Ren 6 Qihai		Ki. 3 Taixi
Ren 4 Guanyuan		

6.8.3 Analgesia During Childbirth

Acupuncture significantly relieves the pain of childbirth. The duration of labor is also significantly reduced. In the case of weakness of uterine contractions acupuncture increases the activity of the uterus. Episiotomy and subsequent suture of the perineum can also be carried out with acupuncture analgesia. Besides the analgesic and mental relaxing effect, improved cooperation of the mother is frequently seen.

In acupuncture for analgesia during childbirth, local points in the area of the lower abdomen or back are combined with important distal points. The distal points Sp.6 Sanyinjiao and Neima, on the inner side of the leg, are needled unilaterally, which does not obstruct the obstetrician. Other distal points of the leg are also used, and electrical stimulation is applied at these points. Electrical stimulation increases the analgesic effect of acupuncture. LI.4 Hegu, on the hand, is repeatedly stimulated by hand. Generally two local points and two distal points on the legs are selected for electrostimulation.

The points Du 20 Baihui, Ex.6 Sishencong and He.7 Shenmen have a strong relaxing and harmonizing effect, so they should be needled at the beginning.

Du 20	Baihui				
Ex.6	Sishencong				
St.29	Guilai	LI.4	Hegu	Sp.6	Sanyinjiao
Ren 4	Guanyuan	He.7	Shenmen	Extra-Neima	
Du 2	Yaoshu			Liv.3	Taichong
Du 6	Jizhong			St.36	Zusanli
GB.21	Jianjing			UB.67	Zhiyin

6.9 Urological Disorders

In chronic inflammation and in functional disturbances of the urogenital organs, acupuncture treatment is very effective. According to traditional Chinese concepts the kidney system, in addition to its renal functions, includes the urogenital functions. In urological disorders a deficiency of the kidney is usually present, accompanied by reduced activity, tiredness, lack of vitality, cold feet, feeling cold in the lumbar region, low immune resistance and lack of libido. In many cases there are infections of the urogenital region. Weakness of willpower and withdrawal from the environment caused by fear are often predominant.

Important points for urological disorders:

- **Sp. 6 Sanyinjiao,** the meeting point of the three Yin channels, spleen, kidney, and liver, is the most important distal point for the urogenital organs.

- **Liv. 3 Taichong,** the Yuan point, is a further important distal point, because the liver channel passes through the genital region.

- **UB. 23 Shenshu** is the Shu point of the kidney. In kidney disturbances the organ can be directly influenced by way of this point.

- **Ren 3 Zhongji** is the Mu point, or alarm point, of the urinary bladder, and as a local point very important in treatment of the urinary bladder.

- **Ren 4 Guanyuan** is an important tonification point for the Yin in the body, especially for the urogenital organs and for the bladder.

- **Ren 6 Qihai** is an important general tonification point, affecting the urogenital system in particular. Moxibustion is very effective in deficiency disturbances.

6.9.1 Pyelonephritis, Urinary Infections, Chronic Glomerulonephritis

In these disorders, according to the traditional classification of symptoms, often kidney Yang deficiency is present. The symptoms caused by inflammation, such as burning, acute pain, and fever, are an expression of an excess or heat disturbance of the urinary bladder. During treatment the kidney must be strengthened with moxibustion. Needle treatment is used in addition to alleviate the acute excess-type symptoms of the urinary bladder. In urinary infections acupuncture is combined with the appropriate medication, to control the acute infection. Acupuncture and moxibustion, because of their immune-enhancing effect, abolish the relapsing character of urinary infections, so that a chronic course can often be avoided.

Points for moxibustion

UB.23	Shenshu	LI.11	Quchi	Ki.7 Fuliu
GB.25	Jingmen			Ki.8 Jiaoxin
Du 4	Mingmen			Sp.6 Sanyinjiao
UB.28	Pangguangshu			Liv.8 Ququan
UB.25	Dachangshu			Ki.3 Taixi
Ren 4	Guanyuan			
Ren 6	Qihai			

Points for acupuncture

Du 20	Baihui			
Ren 3	Zhongji	LI.4	Hegu	Ki.3 Taixi
UB.23	Shenshu	LI.11	Quchi	Liv.3 Taichong
Du 3	Yaoyangguan			Sp.6 Sanyinjiao
				Ki.6 Zhaohai

6.9.2 Prostatitis, Psychogenic Urological Symptoms

In these chronic irritations, according to traditional ideas, a heat and damp disturbance of the kidney and urinary bladder system is present. Acupuncture treatment is especially successful in predominantly psychosomatic conditions, which are resistant to other forms of treatment.

For weakness symptoms moxibustion is indicated in addition with similar points as for pyelonephritis.

Du 20	Baihui				
Ren 3	Zhongji	LI.4	Hegu	Sp.6	Sanyinjiao
Ren 4	Guanyuan			Ki.5	Shuiquan
UB.23	Shenshu			UB.63	Jinmen
UB.28	Pangguangshu				

6.9.3 Enuresis

Enuresis is traditionally ascribed to a weakness of the kidney Qi. There are many possible causes, mostly psychogenic, e.g., anxiety. Treatment with moxibustion strengthens the kidney Qi. Acupuncture with a tonifying technique is indicated in older children or adolescents. In infants moxibustion and laser treatment should be tried.

Points for moxibustion

UB.23	Shenshu			Ki.3	Taixi
UB.28	Pangguangshu	Lu.9	Taiyuan	Liv.3	Taichong
Ren 3	Zhongji			Sp.6	Sanyinjiao
Ren 4	Guanyuan			St.36	Zusanli
Ren 6	Qihai			UB.40	Weizhong
UB.32	Ciliao			UB.67	Zhiyin

Acupuncture

Du 20	Baihui				
Ren 3	Zhongji	He.7	Shenmen	Sp.6	Sanyinjiao
Ren 4	Guanyuan			Ki.3	Taixi
UB.23	Shenshu			St.36	Zusanli

6.10 Skin Disorders

In many skin disorders, such as acne, herpes zoster, psoriasis, and eczema, acupuncture treatment is effective. According to traditional ideas the skin is related to the lung and the large intestine, and therefore skin disorders are treated with points on these channels. Both excess- and deficiency-type conditions should be considered for needle stimulation.

Principles of treatment:

- **Points surrounding the disorder:** the diseased skin area should not be needled, especially the ulcerated region

- **Points on the lung channel** because the skin is related to the lung

- **Sp. 10 Xuehai** because of its anti-allergic properties

- **Du 14 Dazhui and Sp. 6 Sanyinjiao** because of their anti-inflamatory and immune-enhancing effects

- **LI. 11 Quchi** as a homeostatic point and immune-enhancing properties

- **Lu. 9 Taiyuan** is the influential point for the vascular system and is needled in disturbances of blood supply

Besides needling, **laser treatment** has a major role in the therapy of skin disorders. The laser light can be used to radiate skin lesions, for example in herpes simplex and in deficient wound healing. Local and specific distal acupuncture points are also radiated. The exposure time for radiation treatment applied to whole areas of skin is 2 min/cm^2 with a laser power of 2–10 mW. Each acupuncture point is radiated for 20–30 s.

6.10.1 Acne Vulgaris

In the treatment of acne, acupuncture points in the affected area are selected, for example on the face and back. In addition the specific distal points on those channels passing through the affected region are treated. Laser treatment is also effective.

Acne of the face

Du 20 Baihui
St. 3   Juliao   LI. 4   Hegu   St. 36 Zusanli
St. 5   Daying   LI. 11 Quchi   Sp. 10 Xuehai
St. 6   Jiache   Lu. 7   Lieque   Sp. 6   Sanyinjiao
St. 7   Xiaguan   Pe. 4   Ximen
Further local points

Acne of the back

Du 20   Baihui
Du 14   Dazhui   LI. 11 Quchi   UB. 40 Weizhong
Du 12   Shenzhu   Lu. 7   Lieque   UB. 60 Kunlun
UB. 13 Feishu   Sp. 10 Xuehai
Further local points

6.10.2 Leg Ulcers, Deficient Wound Healing

In this case radiation of the skin lesions concerned is surprisingly effective. Within a few days new granulation tissue forms, and lesions that have been present for years start to heal. Besides laser treatment, acupuncture is also effective.

Local points: Points proximal and distal to the ulcer. Points on channels passing through the affected area. Points corresponding to the location of the ulcer on the contralateral side of the body.

General points

Du 20 Baihui   Lu. 9 Taiyuan   Sp. 6   Sanyinjiao
Du 14 Dazhui   Lu. 7 Lieque
                    LI. 11 Quchi

6.10.3 Eczema, Neurodermatitis

According to traditional ideas a Yin deficiency of the lung is present in these conditions. In the treatment of eczema, stimulation of the points on the lung and large intestine channels is effective. Moxibustion of important distal points can also be useful. Changed nutritional habits are essential for the success of treatment.

Du 20 Baihui		
Du 14 Dazhui	LI. 11 Quchi	Sp. 10 Xuehai
Points of the	He. 7 Shenmen	Sp. 6 Sanyinjiao
affected region	LI. 4 Hegu	St. 36 Zusanli

6.10.4 Psoriasis

In psoriasis success can be achieved only with long-term treatment. In most cases two to four cycles of treatment, each of 10–12 sessions, are required. Laser treatment of the affected skin area is very successful.

Du 20 Baihui		
Points of the	LI. 11 Quchi	Sp. 10 Xuehai
affected area	Lu. 5 Chize	Sp. 6 Sanyinjiao
	Lu. 7 Lieque	St. 36 Zusanli

6.10.5 Herpes Simplex

If possible the skin lesions should be radiated with laser light when the first pustules occur. The exposure time should be 2 min/cm^2 with a laser power of 2–10 mW. The distal points for the face, such as LI. 4 Hegu and LI. 11 Quchi, are indicated in addition. In genital herpes Sp. 6 Sanyinjiao and Sp. 10 Xuehai are radiated or needled. After daily treatment for 3–4 days the lesions are usually cured. Laser treatment reduces the relapse rate.

6.11 Disorders of the Sense Organs

In disorders of the sense organs deafness, tinnitus, vertigo, conjunctivitis, and visual deficiency are the major indications. Clinical research from China verifies the high effectiveness of acupuncture treatment in disorders of the sense organs, although the mechanism of effect is still unknown. According to traditional ideas the ear is related to the functional system of the kidney and urinary bladder, while the eye corresponds to the liver and gallbladder. In addition there are close connections between the ear and the Sanjiao channel, which circles round the ear, and stimulation of the distal points of the Sanjiao is highly effective in ear disorders.

6.11.1 Deafness

According to traditional criteria weakness symptoms of the kidney and Sanjiao are generally predominant. Therefore, in addition to acupuncture treatment moxibustion is also indicated.

Du 20	Baihui				
SJ.21	Ermen	SJ.3	Zhongzhu	GB.41	Foot Linqi
SI.19	Tinggong	SJ.5	Waiguan		
GB.2	Tinghui	LI.4	Hegu		
SJ.17	Yifeng	SI.6	Yanglao		
GB.20	Fengchi	SI.3	Houxi		
Du 15	Yamen				

Moxibustion

UB.23	Shenshu	SJ.3	Zhongzhu	Ki.3	Taixi
UB.22	Sanjiaoshu			Ki.7	Fuliu

6.11.2 Tinnitus

Acupuncture is especially indicated when earlier medication has been ineffective. According to traditional ideas either an excess-type disturbance of the liver or gallbladder with a heavy sensation in the head or headache, or a deficiency-type disturbance of the kidney system with typical cold symptoms is present.

Du 20 Baihui
SJ. 21 Ermen   SJ. 3 Zhongzhu   Liv. 3   Taichong
SJ. 17 Yifeng   Liv. 2   Xingjian
GB. 2   Tinghui   GB. 41   Foot Linqi

Moxibustion

UB. 23 Shenshu   SJ. 3 Zhongzhu   Ki. 3 Taixi
Du 4   Mingmen   Lu. 9 Taiyuan   Ki. 7 Fuliu
                                               Sp. 6 Sanyinjiao

6.11.3 Ménière's Syndrome, Dizziness, Motion Sickness, Labyrinthitis

Acupuncture is effective in various types of dizziness. According to traditional ideas a disharmony of Yin and Yang is present, often also a deficiency disturbance of the Sanjiao or the kidney system and an excess of the liver.

Du 20 Baihui
SJ. 21 Ermen   SJ. 3 Zhongzhu   GB. 41 Foot Linqi
SI. 19 Tinggong   SJ. 5 Waiguan   Liv. 3 Taichong
GB. 2   Tinghui   LI. 4 Hegu
                        SI. 6 Yanglao

Moxibustion is indicated for pronounced weakness symptoms.

6.11.4 Chronic Conjunctivitis

In chronic conjunctivitis and in other sorts of irritation of the eye, e.g., intolerance to contact lenses, acupuncture treatment has a good result.

In Chinese medicine these states of irritation are described as "ascending fire of the liver." External climatic influences, such as wind or heat, may also contribute to them.

When points in the area of the orbit are needled, great care must be taken not to injure the eye. Beginners should not needle these points. Distal points on the liver and gallbladder channels, GB.37 Guangming, the Luo point, and Liv.3 Taichong, the Yuan point, are very important.

Du 20	Baihui				
Ex.2	Taiyang	LI.4	Hegu	Liv.3	Taichong
UB.1	Jingming	LI.11	Quchi	GB.37	Guangming
SJ.23	Sizhukong			Sp.6	Sanyinjiao
St.1	Chengqi				
GB.1	Tongziliao				
GB.20	Fengchi				
Du 14	Dazhui				

6.11.5 Vision Deficiency

A deficiency of vision can be caused by many eye disorders. After exhaustion of the standard ophthalmological treatments it is advisable to try acupuncture, because sometimes significant improvements in vision can be achieved.

Du 20	Baihui				
St.1	Chengqi	LI.4	Hegu	GB.37	Guangming
Ex.4	Qiuhou	SI.6	Yanglao	UB.18	Ganshu
UB.2	Zanzhu	LI.5	Yangxi	Sp.6	Sanyinjiao
GB.14	Yangbai	LI.11	Quchi	Liv.3	Taichong
GB.20	Fengchi			St.36	Zusanli
Ex.2	Taiyang				

6.12 Acute Disorders and Emergencies

In many acute disorders, such as fainting, collapse, grand mal epilepsy, and acute pain, acupuncture in addition to the usual emergency treatment is often very effective. For example a patient in an acute attack can be needled while a syringe is prepared for injection of the appropriate drug. In collapse the circulation can be stabilized within seconds. Usually only Jing points that have a direct effect are needled. In acute emergencies, if no needles are available, exceptionally thin disposable cannulae can be used. Acupuncture is also useful for diagnosis in acute emergencies. If a comatose patient does not react to needling, the coma is deep and dangerous.

Principles of treatment:

- Needling and stimulation of **Jing points**
- Needling of specific distal points for fast relief of pain and other symptoms
- Needling of local, spontaneously sensitive, or pressure-sensitive Ah Shi points
- Needling of **Xi-cleft points** corresponding to the affected organs
- Needling of **Du 20 Baihui** with sedative effect

6.12.1 Fainting, Collapse

Du 26 Renzhong

Vigorous manual stimulation of the needles. If no acupuncture needles are available, acupressure with the thumbnail should be tried.

6.12.2 Epileptic Fits, Grand Mal

In an acute attack **Du 26 Renzhong** is needled and vigorously stimulated. Often the attacks are aborted immediately.

6.12.3 Acutely Painful Conditions

In acutely painful conditions, e.g., renal or gallbladder colic, cardiac infarction, or acute abdominal pain, needling of important analgesic points reduces the pain within a short time. Further diagnostic and therapeutic procedures are eased. Important points for acute pain conditions:

LI.4 Hegu on the hand
St.44 Neiting on the foot

These points are vigorously manualy stimulated.

7 Electroacupuncture and Transcutaneous Electrical Nerve Stimulation

B. POMERANZ

7.1 Electroacupuncture, EA

As outlined in Chap. 2, stimulation of high threshold muscle sensory nerves (type II and III muscle afferents) is the basis of AA. Neural messages are then sent to the brain (or spinal cord) where neurochemicals and hormones are released. In ancient times in order to stimulate the nerves, the acupuncture needle was rotated (or jiggled or moved in and out) to create De Qi, a deep aching sensation, with fullness, tingling, and numbness. The failure to achieve De Qi usually meant poor results. As described in Chap. 2, the injection of procaine into the acupuncture point (prior to needle manipulation) abolished AA, proving the importance of activating the nerves. It is interesting to note that procaine injected just under the skin (subcutaneously) did not block acupuncture effects; only deep injections into the muscle were able to do so, thus showing the involvement of deep muscle nerves rather than superficial skin nerves. Recently, microneurography in humans showed that De Qi was mediated by high threshold type II and III muscle nerves (see Chap. 2).

In 1958 when the Chinese were developing methods of acupuncture for surgical anesthesia, they found it inconvenient to have several acupuncturists reaching under the bedsheets to twirl the needles continuously for several hours. Instead they attached flexible wires (via small alligator clips) to the needles and stimulated them electrically. Thus electroacupuncture (EA) was born.

In China in the 1960s, after several years of use for surgical analgesia, EA was introduced into clinical practice, especially for treatment of chronic pain and neurological diseases.

In modern practice in Europe and America, EA allows the practitioner to treat the patient with chronic pain for 15 to 30 min while attending to other patients at the same time in adjacent rooms. Usually 4–8 needles can be stimulated at one time via parallel channels on the stimulator. For example if 6 needles are stimulated, three independent (parallel) channels are used, each channel serving one pair of needles. One pair of needles (and wires) is needed to complete the circuit. Generally the red lead of each pair is positive, and the black lead is negative. Pulses of electricity are applied to the needles in order to stimulate nerves, with the pulse width being from 0.1 to 1.0 ms in duration. (Some stimulators have adjustable pulse width.) More expensive, elaborate stimulators use biphasic pulses (negative followed by positive or vice versa) in order to reduce polarization of each needle due to electrolysis. (The negative pulse cleans the electrode of electrolytes deposited by the preceding positive pulse.) If the pulses are perfectly biphasic, then the net DC current is zero and no polarization occurs. Polarization is a nuisance as it raises the electrode resistance over time, thus reducing the intensity of stimulation. Also, it can cause the needle to break off in the tissue.

Another advantage of biphasic pulses is that the two needles of each pair receive symmetrical stimuli (one needle being the mirror image of the other). Hence the red lead has a positive pulse immediately followed by a negative pulse, while the black lead has a negative pulse followed by a positive pulse. Since negative pulses cause an action potential on the nerve, it is important that both needles in a pair receive negative pulses, which is only possible in a biphasic stimulator. The intensity of stimulation is under the control of an intensity knob. In less expensive stimulators in which biphasic pulses are not perfectly matched (the negative wave is not equal to the positive wave), the negative, black lead will give a stronger needle sensation than the positive, red lead. In order to achieve an optimum effect for AA, the strongest tolerable intensity is required for De Qi (to activate type II and III muscle nerves). If both leads of a pair deliver symmetrical, biphasic pulses then both needles will be optimally stimulated to give De Qi. With less expensive devices however, only one needle of a pair is adequately activated (the needle attached to the black lead).

Generally, muscles begin to contract at the threshold for the largest nerve fibres (e.g., 0.1-ms duration, 5 V, 0.5 mA peak current, assuming a needle resistance of 10 kç). The finer the needle, the higher the resistance; hence, a greater applied voltage will be required to reach threshold. The important parameter in order to produce action potentials is the intensity in terms of coulombs of charge (which is pulse duration in milliseconds multiplied by pulse amplitude in milliamps). Increasing the pulse width lowers the required pulse amplitude to reach threshold. Inexpensive stimulators often do not give a square wave pulse, and thus pulse width does not mean the same thing for all devices. Pulses wider than 1.0 ms do not further enhance nerve activation; they only increase problems due to polarization, electrophoresis and tissue heating, and limit the frequencies of pulses which can be used. To achieve De Qi from type III nerves usually requires stimulus intensities 5 to 10 times threshold levels for muscle contraction (e.g., 25–50 V, 2.5–5 mA, at a pulse width of 0.1 ms). Needles insulated to the tips ensure deep muscle De Qi sensations while minimizing burning sensations from the skin.

Another critical parameter is the pulse frequency (number of stimuli per second, usually expressed as Hertz or Hz). In ancient China the needles were often manually manipulated with a rhythm of 2–4 Hz. For surgical anesthesia in the 1960s 4 Hz was used. Research has shown that 4 Hz releases endorphins and cortisol (see Chap.2). However, conventional TENS is based on frequencies ranging from 50 to 200 Hz (see Sect.7.2 below). Some devices use trains of pulses (bursts instead of continuous pulses) with an internal frequency of 200 Hz and a repetition rate of 4 Hz. Another point to remember is that low frequency stimulation gives individual muscle twitches, while high frequency (anything above 20 Hz) gives tetanic spastic contraction as the muscle has no time to relax between contractions. Originally, trains were used to allow the muscle to relax between bursts and hence make the stimuli more comfortable. However, experience has shown that trains also cause muscle spasms at high intensities, thus preventing the achievement of De Qi which is so important for producing endorphin analgesia. Hence, 4 Hz without trains is best for obtaining De Qi. Some devices provide a continuously varying frequency pattern called "dense dispersed" in order to overcome habituation to monotonous stimulation. These devices sweep from 4 Hz (dispersed) to 200 Hz (dense) in a continually varying cycle. Unfortunately, this doesn't allow the strong intense stimulation (required for De Qi) as the intensity is limited by the muscle spasms caused by the 200-Hz part of the cycle. Also this type of antihabituation is not effective in overcoming habituation (see section 7.4). To summarize: De Qi is only achievable at 2–4 Hz, while high frequency or trains (or dense dispersed) must be avoided as these cause muscle spasms and prevent the De Qi.

As stated above, strong stimulation is needed to release cortisone and endorphins (type III afferents must be activated to produce De Qi). Small-diameter afferent nerve fibres (type III) require considerable current (high intensity) for activation. Hence the intensity must be raised to 5 or 10 times the threshold level for muscle contraction. Because contractions often become vigorous, the stimulus intensity must be raised gradually. The patient has to be reassured that the procedure is not harmful, dangerous, or frankly painful. De Qi is a mild, pleasant, ache which is easily tolerated by most patients. However, some patients are afraid of electricity; they may also fear the muscle contractions and must be slowly introduced to the procedure. On the first office visit, the intensity should be raised in steps (say every 5 min for 30 min) until intense muscle contractions are observed. Sometimes the second treatment session is the best time to introduce strong stimulation. Be aware that different regions of the body have different sensitivities, e.g., the face is extremely sensitive and much lower currents must be used. Also, instead of deep sensations and muscle contractions typical of De Qi, the sensations on the face tend to be sharp and burning due to skin nerves being activated. Thus, when adjusting the intensity for face needles, raise the voltage current levels very slowly and cautiously. Also be sure to pair the needles for each stimulator channel in body regions of equal sensitivity (e.g., do not place one needle on the face and the other paired needle on the hand). Note that the United States Food and Drug Administration (FDA) does not permit use of electrical stimulation around the head or ears.

There is very little danger from EA for several reasons. The devices are battery operated, so stray currents from the lines are avoided. The currents used are well below the levels which can affect the heart. The American Association for Medical Instrumentation (AAMI) recommends safety levels to be below 25 microcoulombs per pulse if electrodes are placed across the heart (i.e., arm to arm). This is equivalent to 25 mA at 1.0 ms or 250 mA at 0.1 ms pulse width. De Qi is usually achieved with 2.5–5 mA at 0.1 ms pulse width, which is well below AAMI safety levels. However, patients with heart pacemakers should not use EA. Also stimulation over the neck region is to be avoided to prevent laryngospasm. Finally, strong stimulation in spastic muscles (Ah Shi points, trigger points, tender spots) could aggravate the spasms and hence should be avoided.

A major advantage of EA is that the margin of error in needle placement for EA is greater than for manual therapy, and thus less accurate needle placement is required (to obtain De Qi with manual needling requires precise placement into the acupoint; if the needle misses the mark during EA, the current spreads out from the needle and may reach the nerve up to several millimetres away). Unfortunately, there have been no controlled studies to see whether EA works better than manual needle twirling.

Research on animals and human volunteers reveals that it takes 20–30 min for endorphinergic analgesia to build up, and typically the preparation for surgical "anesthesia" takes 30 min of stimulation. At the end of 20–30 min of EA therapy, all intensity knobs should be turned down to zero, and the leads disconnected from the patient. The device should not be switched off while the patient is still connected as there might be "surge" shocks at the off.

If one is treating according to traditional Chinese medicine, EA intensities should be determined by the requirement to sedate or to tonify. When sedating use high intensity (5 to 10 times threshold) to achieve De Qi; when tonifying use low intensity (just above threshold). Generally, pain therapy requires sedation, but in some patients who are debilitated by chronic pain, tonification may be indicated.

7.2 Transcutaneous Electrical Nerve Stimulation, TENS

With TENS, nerve stimulation can be given without the use of needles. For this purpose small flexible electrode pads consisting of electroconductive carbon-filled vinyl sheets (usually 2 cm × 3 cm) are attached to the skin over the acupuncture point (one pair of electrodes for each stimulator channel). The current/voltage intensity is turned up until the nerves under the skin are activated transcutaneously. For TENS higher currents/voltages are used than for EA because the current density is less with pads than with needles. This is the case for two reasons: first the current with pads is spread over a wide area (6 cm^2) while the current with needles is concentrated into 1 mm^2, and second the needles, which penetrate the skin, bring about a lower skin resistance allowing for deeper penetration of the current. For TENS to achieve deep penetration to the muscle nerves the following conditions are required:

1. Good electrode contact with the skin (uneven contact could result in skin burns at the edges of the pad due to high current densities). Adhesive tape or velcro straps are useful here.
2. Proper pad to skin electrolyte contact (EKG gels are usually not as good as Karaya, which is a self-adhesive conductive material first invented for colostomy bags). A poor interface requires large voltages (above 200 V) to achieve the current levels needed to activate deep muscle nerves.
3. Use of square pulse shapes with a fast rise time to overcome the capacitance of the skin (less than 5 ms is desirable).
4. Antipolarization biphasic pulses (described above for EA).
5. High stimulus intensities (up to 25 mA, 250 V, assuming electrode resistance of 10 kΩ and 1 ms pulses; with a 0.1-ms pulse width, larger pulse amplitudes are used).
6. Large electrode pads (6 cm^2) lower the skin resistance and keep the current densities at the skin below painful levels, while allowing large enough currents to reach the muscle where the type III nerves are situated. If pads are too large, however, current density will drop too low, and deep muscle nerves will not be activated.

7. The best devices use constant current sources, to overcome the variations in skin-electrode resistance which occur from time to time during a 30-min therapy session. They also ensure square pulses by overcoming the skin capacitance.

TENS has advantages and disadvantages when compared with EA. Advantages include the omission of needles which have certain risks such as infection, and pneumothorax. Many patients have a fear of needles, and prefer TENS. Perhaps the most compelling reason for TENS is the ease of use: not as much precision is required in the placement of pads over acupuncture points as the current will find its way to the nerve, given the large areas covered by the pad. Ease of use makes TENS especially attractive for novices who are uncertain of point location, depth of penetration or angle of the needle trajectory. Moreover, home use (self-administered by the patient) is possible with TENS. If employed 30 min a day on a daily basis cumulative effects occur which are more powerful than office treatments twice a week.

The disadvantages of TENS must also be considered. Most TENS devices cannot achieve De Qi sensations even at high current intensities. This is because the pulse shapes they emit cause burning and cutting sensations from skin nerves instead of deep aching De Qi from type III muscle afferents. Even with proper TENS devices, some patients do not like strong stimulation (with accompanying strong muscle contractions), and hence they never achieve the benefit of stimulating type III muscle afferents (De Qi). Remember that De Qi is the goal of EA for treating pain, and with TENS this is only achieved with strong stimulation. Before first choosing any TENS device the clinician is well advised to try out several units on himself/herself to determine whether De Qi sensations can be elicited without accompanying burning sensations from the skin (an easy location to perform this test is on Li. 4).

Another disadvantage of TENS is the difficulty of applying TENS pads to points on the face, ears, scalp, nose, etc. For this purpose some machines have hand-held, pencil-shaped probes with saline-soaked cotton or metal tips (wet cotton is preferred as it makes better contact). Generally one gives 30 s of treatment at each point. The patient completes the circuit by holding the red lead connected to a stainless steel cylinder which makes contact with the moist palm of the hand. Most of these devices with stimulating probes suffer from the disadvantage that small areas of the skin are contacted, requiring a high current density at the skin to achieve sufficient current at the deep muscle nerve, leading to burning sensations from the skin instead of De Qi from the muscle. While probes may be useful over acupoints with superficial nerves (e.g., ear, some face points, fingertips, etc.), they are useless for body acupuncture. The proof of this is the fact that neither De Qi nor deep muscle contractions are experienced with probe stimulators used on body acupoints. Indeed, many probe stimulators only deliver maximum currents of 600 μA, which means that it is practically impossible for current to reach deep muscle nerves. Another disadvantage of these probe devices is the need to be very accurate with placement of the tip. Given the small currents/voltage, the chance of hitting the nerve is minimal unless the probe is exactly placed (over a low resistance acupoint and close to the nerve). The high current density will usually cause skin burning before deep nerve sensations, and hence direct hits over the nerve are necessary. The inconvenience of holding the probe prevents the therapist from giving 20–30 min of therapy, or from stimulating 6–8 acupoints simultaneously. Thus pads are far superior to probes for TENS.

7.3 Acupuncture-like TENS Differs from Conventional TENS

The use of low-frequency, high-intensity TENS to stimulate acupuncture points (to produce De Qi) is called acupuncture-like TENS and should not be confused with conventional TENS which uses high frequency, low intensity stimulation. These two methods differ in several important respects. Conventional TENS was developed in the early 1970s as a result of the Gate Theory of pain (see Chap. 2). For analgesia to occur according to this theory, large-diameter afferents (type I muscle afferents and A beta skin afferents) are stimulated at low intensity and high frequency in the same dermatome (or myotome or segment) as the site of the pain. This releases GABA to cause presynaptic inhibition of adjacent pain fibres (small-diameter A delta and C afferents which carry the pain message). This presynaptic inhibition prevents pain messages from reaching the spinal cord transmission neurons. This form of analgesia starts within 100 ms of TENS stimulation and disappears within seconds of turning off the machine. Hence, conventional TENS must typically be used throughout the day to obtain sustained analgesia. Acupuncture-like TENS can be given as little as twice a week with lasting effects because of endorphin release (see below).

An essential feature of acupuncture-like TENS is the use of strong stimulation to produce De Qi (this is similar to low-frequency EA using needles). Small-diameter, high-threshold fibres are activated. To achieve De Qi in type III muscle afferents usually requires 5–10 times the current (voltage) needed to stimulate low-threshold type I fibres. In practical terms De Qi occurs with current (voltage) stimulation which is 5–10 times the threshold value for muscle contraction. Intensity is kept just below frank pain so that a pleasant, mild, aching sensation is felt. Although weaker stimulation by conventional TENS can release some endorphins, the stronger intensities of acupuncture-like TENS recruit type III fibres, causing a greater effect. Unfortunately, many clinicians hesitate to use strong stimulation for fear of hurting their patient. Because much coaxing is needed to raise the intensities, many therapists fail to achieve De Qi, and their treatments become conventional TENS (where only large-fiber stimulation occurs). As stated above, an important problem arises because many TENS devices do not have appropriate pulse characteristics to achieve De Qi and consequently burning at the skin often occurs at voltages (currents) below those needed to activate type III muscle nerves. Most TENS devices are designed for conventional TENS purposes (large-fibre stimulation). A few TENS devices, however, can achieve De Qi, and acupuncture-like TENS becomes possible.

Conventional TENS is mainly segmental in nature, not involving pituitary mechanisms. In contrast, acupuncture-like TENS combines segmental and nonsegmental effects: it involves brain stem, pituitary plus segmental mechanisms via endorphins and serotonin (see Fig. 2, Chap. 1 for similarities to low frequency EA). Acupuncture-like TENS involves stimulation of mapped acupuncture points, which helps to locate type III afferents. Also acupuncture-like TENS usually takes 20–30 min to reach a maximum effect, and the analgesia outlasts the therapy by several hours (or days). Hence continuous treatment throughout the day is not required with acupuncture-like TENS, making it superior to conventional TENS.

The major differences between conventional TENS and acupuncture-like TENS are summarized in Table 7.1.

Table 7.1. Comparison of the two methods for TENS

Conventional TENS	Acupuncture-like TENS
High frequency, low intensity, Gate Theory	Low frequency, high intensity, De Qi
Low intensity activates large muscle (type I) and large skin ($A\beta$) nerves for Gate effect	High intensity pulses produce De Qi via small muscle (type III) nerves to release endorphins
Segmental effects based on Gate Theory: large diameter fibers inhibit pain from small fibers	Nonsegmental and segmental effects: small fibers act on three sites: spine, brainstem and pituitary
High intensity of most TENS devices causes burning from skin but no De Qi from muscle	High intensity of some TENS devices activates small muscle (type III) nerves producing De Qi
Pads are placed near the site of pain as large diameter fibers are widely distributed	Pads placed on acupuncture points as these are over small diameter afferent nerves (type III) in muscle
High frequency (50–200 Hz) produces best presynaptic inhibition at low intensity (for Gate) but produces spasms at high intensity	Low frequency (2–4 Hz) produces no muscle spasm at high intensity and hence allows strong stimulation needed for De Qi
Trains maximize comfort of low intensity, high frequency stimulation	Trains cause muscle spasms at high intensity and do not permit adequate intensities for De Qi
Analgesia has rapid onset and short duration requiring continuous treatment all day long	Analgesia has slow onset and long duration: needs only 30 min of therapy for prolonged effects
Tolerance develops from continuous therapy	No tolerance from short, 30 min, treatments

Lower frequency stimulation is used (4 Hz) to achieve De Qi, as high frequency causes muscle spasms at the intensity needed to produce the aching sensation. For conventional TENS, high frequency is used (50–200 Hz) as this causes the optimum presynaptic inhibition through the Gate mechanism, but De Qi is not achieved because muscle spasms prevent the use of sufficient intensity to activate type III nerves.

There are many TENS devices commercially available, but only a few are suitable for acupuncture-like TENS (caviat emptor; buyer beware).

On the whole, acupuncture-like TENS is superior to conventional TENS because it produces prolonged analgesia and thus does not have to be worn continuously by the patient. One 30-min treatment session a day (or twice a week) is sufficient therapy using acupuncture like TENS for chronic pain. This is similar to the experience with EA or manual acupuncture in which prolonged effects are achieved.

7.4 Habituation to Monotonous Stimuli

Continuous, repetitive, monotonous stimulation by TENS or EA causes habituation of the nervous system. Hence, 30-min treatments are wasted, since only the first few minutes of stimuli are effective. The use of random switching of stimuli among six different electrodes overcomes this problem, as the brain perceives each site as a novel stimulus. This method of stimulation is called dishabituation (or heterosynaptic facilitation by some neurophysiologists).

8 Traditional Chinese Syndromes: The Diagnosis of Chinese Medicine

G. STUX

Traditional Chinese Medicine has a functional nosology based on disturbances of the five Zang organs (lung, heart, spleen, liver, kidney) and the six Fu organs (large intestine, small instestine, stomach, gallbladder and urinary bladder).

It categorizes these functional disturbances with the help of the eight diagnostic criteria (Ba gang), namely Yin and Yang, interior and exterior, deficiency and excess, cold and heat in a process of the four examinations: visual observation, listening and smelling, questioning and physical examination (see chapter 3.4). From this comes about 50 clearly defined differentiations called "Traditional Chinese Syndromes" or "Patterns of Disharmony." The diagnostic identification of these syndromes is essential for the treatment of disease, particularly chronic conditions.

Deficiency or excess disturbances of Qi, Blood, or of the Yang or Yin aspects of the Zang organs are differentiated. On the organ level, Yin and Yang functions can be categorized:

- The *Yang function of organs*, for example digestion or respiration is the active and dynamic potential. The warming function in the body is also attributed to Yang. On the mental level, aggression and creativity are considered Yang properties.
- *Yin on the organ level* means structure and the functional potential. The Ying nourishes and moistens the organ and controlls the normal function of Yang. When Yin is deficient, Yang and heat become overactive. Body-fluids are dependent on the Yin aspect of the organs. Identity and mental receptivity are Yin potentials. Aging may be considered dependent on the deminishing of the Yin. When Yin is weakened, aging is accelerated. Cancer, rheumatoid arthritis, tuberculosis and Aids are major exam-

ples where, according to traditional Chinese medicine, Yin-deficiency is dominant.

A third major pattern of disturbance is *stagnation* which can occur especially in the liver, as well in the blood and in the channels.

8.1 Major Patterns of Disturbances

Deficiency of Qi

Etiology: Hyperactivity, overwork, mental stress, long illness, diet, old age.

Symptoms: Hypofunction of organs, (i.e. digestion or respiration) fatigue, lethargy, hypoactivity, pale face, low voice, dislike to speak, shortness of breath, sweating after exhaustion, mental depression, deficient immune responce.

Tongue: pale; Pulse: deficient, weak, empty.

Principles of treatment: Tonify the Qi.

St.36	Zusanli	Sp.6	Sanyinjiao
Ren 6	Qihai	Ren 4	Guanyuan
UB.20	Pishu		

Deficiency of Yang

Symptoms: Symptoms similar to deficiency of Qi but more severe, plus cold symptoms such as aversion to cold, feeling of coldness in the body, cold hands and feet, cold sweating, dizziness. Many patients suffer from hypotension, deficient immune reponce, and they have often respiratory or urogenital infections.

Tongue: white coating; Pulse: weak and slow.

Principles of treatment: Tonify the Qi, warm the Yang

The points are similar to the Qi-tonifying points, moxibustion is used intensively in addition to needling.

Stagnation of Qi

Stagnation of the flow of Qi in organs or channels
Etiology: External climatic influences, diet, emotional factors, i.e.
anger and rage, physical trauma, deficiency of Qi.
Symptoms: Pain and distension, which may change intensity and
location, particularly in the chest, abdomen and limbs, feeling of
stagnation in the body, local edema;
Tongue: purplish; Pulse: wiry, tight.
Principles of treatment: Activate the flow of the Qi.

Liv.3	Taichong	LI.4	Hegu
LI.11	Quchi	St.36	Zusanli
SJ.6	Zhigou	Gb.34	Yanglingquan

Deficiency of Yin

Etiology: Exhaution after a long illness (late stage of chronic disorders), excessive work for a long period, mental stress, excessive
alcohol, excessive sexual activity; Repletion of Yin and fluids in
chronic disease.
Symptoms: Extreme fatigue, feeling of weakness, pale lusterless
face, restlessness, nervousness, agitation, insomnia, much dream-
ing, heat sensation on palms and soles, dry mouth, dry nose, dry
eyes, night sweating.
Tongue: red, with thin coat; Pulse: thin, rapid.
Yin deficiency causes overactive Yang functions, dryness and inter-
nal heat (Yin unable to controll Yang).
Principles of treatment: nourish Yin, sedate Yang, eliminate the
heat:
– Behavioral: resting, relaxation, receptive activities, regeneration.
– Nutritional: pear, plum, dates, waterchesnut, mulberry, coconut
  fluid, watermelon, cucumber, tomato, celery, honey.
– Acupuncture and Moxibustion:
  Kidney: Ki.3, UB.23, Ki.7 [Ki.6, He.6, Lu.5]
  Lung: UB.13, UB.43, Lu.9 [Sp.6, Pe.7]
  Liver: UB.18, Gb.37, Ki.6 [Liv.3, Liv.2]
  Heart: UB.15, He.7, He.3

Deficiency of Blood

Etiology: Loss of blood, deficient spleen Qi, poor nutrition.
Symptoms: Pale, lusterless face and lips, loss of weight, fatigue, dry skin, dizziness, hypotension, blurred vision, sleep disturbances, paresthesia and temor of the limbs and cold limbs.

Following, the different syndromes of the Zang organs are presented.

8.2 Syndromes of the Five Zang Organs

Syndromes of the Lung

The lung tends to develop deficiency-type disturbances, the most common being deficiency of the lung Qi. External pathogenic influences commonly cause deficient lung, allowing wind-cold or wind-heat invasion at different levels. In severe cases phlegm can develop and obstructs the lung. These syndromes are very common, and known in western medicine as infections of the respiratory organs.

Deficiency of lung Yin is a chronic condition, characterized by injury of the Yin, the structuring substance of the lung, allowing excessive Yang and heat symptoms to dominate.
The syndromes of the lung include:

1. Deficiency of Lung Qi	*Fei Qi Xu*
2. Deficiency of Lung Yin	*Fei Yin Xu*
3. Wind-cold affects the Lung	*Feng Han Su Fei*
4. Wind-heat affects the Lung	*Feng Re Fan Fei*
5. Phlegm obstructs the Lung	*Tan Shi Zu Fei*

Syndromes of the Kidney

The kidney can develop a wide range of deficiency syndromes. Deficiency of kidney Yang is most common and characterized by coldness symptoms; it is common in western countries and is the basis for urinary infections.

Deficiency of the kidney can be the foundation of other disturbances of Zang organs, especially lung, spleen or liver.
The syndromes of the kidney include:

1. Deficiency of Kidney Yang   *Shen Yang Xu*
2. Deficiency of Kidney Qi   *Shen Qi Xu*
3. Deficiency of Kidney Yin   *Shen Yin Xu*
4. Deficiency of Kidney Jing   *Shen Jing Xu*

Syndromes of the Liver

The liver, according to Chinese medicine, is responsible for the flow of Qi and blood. Most clinical disturbances of the liver are characterized by stagnation and excess. In chronic cases one may see deficiency of liver Yin or in rare cases deficiency of liver blood. Patients with liver disturbances may shift from Yang excess to deficiency symptoms, for example from excessive headache or migraine to periods of weakness and exhaustion.
The major syndromes of the liver and gallbladder include:

1. Stagnation of Liver Qi   *Gan Qi Yu Jie*
2. Rising Liver Yang   *Gan Yang Shang Kang*
3. Rising Liver Fire   *Gan Shang Yan*
4. Liver-wind moving internally   *Gan Feng Nei Dong*
5. Deficiency of Liver Yin   *Gan Yin Xu*
6. Deficiency of Liver Blood   *Gan Xue Xu*
7. Cold stagnation in the Liver channel   *Han Zhi Gan Mai*
8. Damp-heat in the Liver and Gallbladder   *Gan Dan Shi Re*
9. Deficiency of the Gallbladder and   *Dan Yu Tan Rao*
   Stagnation of Phlegm

Syndromes of the Spleen

Spleen disturbances are characterized by deficiency of Qi or Yang. External influences such as damp, cold or heat, also cold food may cause deficient spleen. Spleen deficiency can cause excess with stasis of Qi in the stomach.

The syndromes of the spleen and stomach include:

1. Deficiency of Spleen Qi   *Pi Qi Xu*
2. Deficiency of Spleen Yang   *Pi Yang Xu*
3. Damp-cold in the Spleen   *Han Shi Kun Pi*
4. Damp-heat in the Spleen   *Pi Yun Shi Re*
5. Phlegm affecting the head   *Tan Zhou Shang Rao*
6. Rising Stomach Fire   *Wei Huo Shang Sheng*
7. Deficiency of the Stomach Yin   *Wei Yin Xu*

Syndromes of the Heart

The heart, according to Chinese medicine, regulates the flow of blood and is also responsible for mental functions. Heart syndromes may be characterized by excess and heat causing nervousness, restlessness, palpitation, and feeling of tension. Heart syndromes may also be caused by deficiency of Qi, Yang, or blood. Heart syndromes are often combined with syndromes of the spleen or kidney. The syndromes of the heart include:

1. Stagnation of Heart Blood   *Xin Xue Yu*
2. Deficiency of Heart Qi   *Xin Qi Xu*
3. Deficiency of Heart Yang   *Xin Yang Xu*
4. Rising Heart Fire   *Xin Huo Shang Yang*
5. Deficiency of Heart Blood   *Xin Xue Xu*
6. Deficiency of Heart Yin   *Xin Yin Xu*

There are 8 Chinese syndromes which are often found in daily clinical practice. Here they are described with etiology, symptomatology, acupuncture treatment, and are related to the diagnosis of western medicine.

8.3 The Most Frequent Syndromes

Deficiency of Lung Qi

Etiology: Exhaustion of energy, chronic diseases of another organ (e. g., spleen or kidney) external pathogenic factors of long duration, old age, exposure to smoke, dust, nicotine, allergies, etc.

Significance: Deficiency of lung Qi is a frequent syndrome and is the basis of many disorders of the lung and the respiratory tract. It often occurs together with deficiency of lung yin, or with cold or heat affecting the lung. It may occur with deficiency disturbances of kidney or spleen.

Western diagnosis: Suspectibility to infections of the respiratory system, including chronic common cold, emphysema, chronic bronchitis, asthma, influenza, allergies.

Symptoms: Weak cough, spastic cough and dyspnea, weak voice, reluctance to speak, shortness of breath after exertion, frequent daytime sweating, aversion to wind, lowered resistance, susceptibility to infection, sensitivity to weather and acute shortness of breath in extreme cases.

Tongue: soft and pale with white coating;

Pulse: weak and fine, dominent on the "cun" position.

Treatment: Principles of treatment is to tonify lung Qi and tonify related organs (spleen, stomach, kidney), treatment with acupuncture and moxibustion.

- UB. 13 Feishu – Shu point of the lung
- Lu. 1 Zhongfu – Mu point of the lung
- Lu. 9 Taiyuan – tonifies the lung Qi
- Lu. 10 Yuji – eliminates pathogenic factors, especially heat
- LI. 11 Quchi – tonifies the large intestine
- Du 14 Dazhui – regulates Yang and Qi, and eliminates pathogenic factors
- Ren 17 Shanzhong – influential point for the respiratory system
- Ren 6 Qihai – tonifies the Qi in general
- St. 36 Zusanli – tonifies the Yang and Qi by the way of tonifying its mother

Deficiency of Spleen Qi

Etiology: Irregular or inadequate absorption of food, malnutrition, overexertion and overwork, constitutional weakness of the digestive organs, chronic diseases.

Significance: Deficiency of spleen Qi is a frequently seen syndrome, especially with aging. This syndrome can be the basis for various other deficiency syndromes such as kidney, and lung. Deficiency of spleen Qi may be subcategorized as "sinking spleen Qi" causing organ prolapses and "spleen not controlling blood" causing purpura and uterine bleeding.

Western diagnosis: Maldigestion, malabsorbtion, anorexia, anemia, diarrhea, gastroenteritis, uterine bleeding.

Symptoms: Lack of appetite, incomplete digestion, loose stool with undigested particles of food, or diarrhea, flatulence, feeling of repletion, pressure sensation in the abdomen, improves after massage, fatigue, weakness, lack of strength, pale, yellowish face, edema of the extremities, soft, unshaped stool, prolapse of uterus and anus, gastroptose, muscle atrophy, lack of strength of the extremities, stool with blood, hypermenorrhea, extravasations; if long-lasting anemia can develop;

Pulse: slow and weak;

Tongue: pale, swollen tongue, with white coat.

Treatment: Principles of treatment is to strengthen the spleen Qi and tonify with moxibustion.

- Liv. 13 Zangmen – influential point for the Zang organs
- UB. 20 Pishu – Shu point of the spleen, benefits spleen
- Ren 12 Zhongwan – tonifies spleen and stomach
- Sp. 6 Sanyinjiao – tonifies spleen
- Sp. 3 Taibai – tonifies spleen
- St. 36 Zusanli – regulates the stomach, tonifies spleen Qi

Deficiency of Spleen Yang

Etiology: Secondary to chronic deficiency of spleen Qi, raw, cold food, excessive sugar consumption and secondary to Yang deficiency of kidney.

Significance: Close relation to deficiency of spleen Qi. Deficiency of spleen Yang is a more severe form of deficiency of spleen Qi, with the additional of cold symptoms. This syndrome is often associated with deficiency of stomach Yang. Deficiency of spleen Yang may lead to a deficient kidney Yang.

Western diagnosis: chronic maldigestion, malabsorbtion, anemia, acute and chronic gastroenteritis, diarrhea.

Symptoms: Cold symptoms including feeling cold and pain in the abdominal region, cold extremities, feeling of cold in the body, relief of the symptoms by pressure and warmth, watery diarrhea with particles of undigested food, edema in the extremities, aching pain in the abdomen, heavy feeling of the limbs and body, weakness, tiredness.

Tongue: pale, watery or slippery coat flabby;

Pulse: deep, weak, slowly.

Treatment: Principles of treatment is to strengthen and warm the Yang of spleen and stomach, eliminate cold; treatment is with acupuncture and moxibustion

– St. 36 Zusanli – tonifies stomach and spleen Qi
– Sp. 6 Sanyinjiao – tonifies spleen
– UB. 20 Pishu – Shu point of the spleen, benefits spleen
– UB. 21 Weishu – Shu point of the stomach
– Ren 12 Zhongwan – Mu point of the stomach, tonifies spleen and stomach
– UB. 23 Shenshu – Shu point of the kidney, strengthens the kidney Qi
– Ren 4 Guanyuan – nourishes Yin, strengthens Yuan source Qi

Deficiency of Kidney Qi

Etiology: Physical exhaustion, constitution, age, mental stress, occuring after chronic disease, excessive sexual activity, many childbirth, secondary to deficient lung Qi.

Significance: special manifestation of deficiency of kidney Yang with less pronounced deficiency and without cold symptoms.

Western diagnosis: Chronic urinary infections, nephritis, sexual disturbances such as frigidity and lack of libido, depression, exhaustion-syndrome, functional syndromes.

Symptoms: Tiredness, lack of energy, depression, fear, hypoactivity, pale, occasionally greyish skin, weakness and soreness in the lumbar region, incontinence, enuresis, – deafness, asthma, chronic cough, (due to failure of kidney to root the Qi of the lung).

Tongue: pale with white coat;

Pulse: deep, weak.

The symptoms are similar to those of deficiency of kidney Yang, but without cold symptoms.

Treatment: Principles of treatment is to strengthen the kidney Qi, combining acupuncture and moxibustion.

- UB.23 Shenshu – Shu point of the kidney, tonifies kidney
- Du 4 Mingmen – strengthen the kidney Qi and Yuan Qi
- Ren 4 Guanyuan – strengthen the Yuan Qi
- Ren 6 Qihai – general tonification point for Qi, Yang and Yuan Qi
- Ki.3 Taixi – Yuan point, strengthens the Yin
- Sp.6 Sanyinjiao – tonifies spleen and kidney, strengthens the Yin
- St.36 Zusanli – general tonification point
- Treatment is similar to that of deficient kidney Yang

Deficiency of Kidney Yang

Etiology: Physical exhaustion, constitutional weakness, old age, mental stress, fear, influence of cold for a long period, chronic diseases of long duration, excessive sexual activity, many childbirths. Deficiency of kidney Qi and Yang is physiological in old age.

Significance: Yang deficiency leads to cold symptoms, reduced mental activity and withdrawal from the environment; Often in combination with other deficient organs such as heart, spleen, and lung. Deficiency of kidney Yang occurs often in old age and in women. Patients with chronic urinary infections suffer on this syndrome, which is seen as cause for low immune resistance.

Western diagnosis: Chronic urinary infections, nephritis, glomerulonephritis, prostatitis, uretritis, sexual disturbances such as frigidity and impotence, depression, fear conditions chronic lumbago, sciatica, degenerative joint disorders, rheumatoid arthritis, hypothyroidism, deafness.

Symptoms: Pale, greyish face, low drive, tiredness, hypoactivity, depressed mood or depression, withdrawal from the environment, fear; coldness symptoms including sensitivity to cold, frequent shivering, cold limbs and sometimes feeling of coldness in the whole body; impotence in men, frigidity in women; feeling of coldness, weakness, or stiffness in the lumbar region, chronic low back pain, urine clear and copious, nykturia, incontinence, irritation of prostate, amenorrhea, disturbances of fertility, deafness, dizziness, tinnitus, morning diarrhea. The symptoms are similar to those of deficiency of kidney Qi but with additional cold symptoms.

Tongue: pale, swollen, with white coat;

Pulse: deep, weak.

Treatment: Principles of treatment is to strengthen and warm the Yang; warm the kidney Yang with moxibustion.

- UB.23 Shenshu – Shu point of the kidney, tonifies kidney
- GB.25 Jingmen – Mu point of the kidney
- Du 4 Mingmen – strengthens the kidney Qi
- Ren 4 Guanyuan – strengthens the Yuan Qi
- Ki.3 Taixi – Yuan point, strengthens the Yin and Yang of the kidney
- Ki.7 Fuliu – tonification point of the kidney
- Ren 6 Qihai – general tonification point for Qi, Yang and Yuan Qi
- Sp.6 Sanyinjiao – tonifies kidney
- St.36 Zusanli – general tonification point
- Lu.9 Taiyuan – tonification point of the lung Qi
- LI.11 Quchi – tonification point of the large intestine

Deficiency of Liver Yin

Etiology: Exhaustion after emotional (i.e., especially anger) or physical excessive stress, after chronic diseases, old age.

Significance: If the liver Yin is deficient, the liver Yang or liver fire are rising uncontrolled. Deficiency of liver Yin is often secondary to depression of liver Qi by rising of liver fire or of liver Yang. Deficiency of liver Yin is usually combined with deficiency of the kidney Yin.

Western diagnosis: Hypertension, chronic fatigue syndrome, chronic conjunctivitis, excessive alkohol.

Symptoms: Fatigue, weakness, red face and cheeks, hot palms and soles, mild pain or burning sensation in the costal region, dry throat and mouth, menstrual disorders, feeling of heat, nervousness, restlessness, dizziness, dry eyes, visual disturbances, mental depression;

Tongue: reddish with little fluid or dry.

Treatment: Principles of treatment is to nourish liver Yin

UB.18 Ganshu – Shu point of the liver

Liv.3 Taichong – harmonizes the liver

Liv.2 Xingjian – for liver fire

Sp.6 Sanyinjiao – strengthens the Yin

UB.23 Shenshu – Shu point of the kidney

Ki.3 Taixi – Yuan point of the kidney, strengthens the Yin and Yang

He.7 Shenmen – sedates the heart

Rising Liver Yang

Etiology: Constitution (choleric temper), excessive alcohol.

Significance: The rising liver Yang is an unbalance between Yin and Yang functions of the liver: liver Yang is in excess, liver Yin is weak, unable to controll the Yang. The uncontrolled Yang rises to the chest and head. In severe and chronic cases it might change into rising liver fire. Usually it is combined with deficiency of the kidney and liver Yin.

Western diagnosis: Migraine, chronic conjunctivitis, glaucoma, hypertension, irritability, restlessness, excitation, rage, anger insomnia.

Symptoms: Headache or feeling of pressure in head, red eyes, flushing, tinnitus, dizziness, visual disturbances, twitching of eye, fullness in the head or chest, insomnia, dryness in mouth and throat, muscle tension, weakness in the lumbar region;

Tongue: red;

Pulse: wiry, thin and rapid.

Treatment: Principles of treatment is to strengthen the liver Yin and harmonize the liver Yang.

Liv.3 Taichong – harmonizes the liver
UB.18 Ganshu – Shu point of the liver
UB.23 Shenshu – Shu point of the kidney
Ki.3 Taixi – strengthens the Yin, Yuan point of the kidney
GB.20 Fengchi – regulates the fire and the Yang of the head
Du 20 Baihui – regulates and harmonizes the Yang of the head
Liv.2 Xingjian – sedates the liver Yang and especially the five in conditions of pronounced symptom

Stagnation of Heart Blood

Etiology: Emotional tension leads to stagnation of Qi and this might lead also to stagnation of blood (Qi and blood are flowing together). Excessive physical activity and mental stress leads to exhaustion and deficiency of Qi causing stasis of blood. Deficient phycical activity leads to stasis of Qi and blood. "Yang deficiency" means, that blood is flowing stagnantly through the heart, so that stasis of blood is occuring.

Significance: Stagnation of heart blood is often related with two common heart deficiency syndromes deficiency of heart Qi or deficiency of heart Yang. The most common heart diseases are based on these three syndromes. May also relate with phlegm disturbances of the heart.

Western diagnosis: Angina pectoris, coronary heart disease, myocardial infarction.

Symptoms: Pain and/or twitches in the chest, pain on the medial side of the left arm, vigorous palpitation, tachycardia, short breath, feeling tightness and tension in the chest, cold extremities and in severe cases, cyanosis of the lips;

Pulse: choppy and excessive;

Tongue: darkred or purple spots on the tongue.

Treatment: Principles of treatment is to eliminate the stagnation and to promote the flow of Qi and blood.

In acute phase:
Pe. 4 Ximen – Xi point of the pericardium
He. 6 Yinxi – Xi point of the heart
Pe. 6 Neiguan – harmonizes the Qi and Yang
Ren 14 Juque – Mu point of the heart
Ren 17 Shanzhong – Mu point of the pericardium
Liv. 3 Taichong – promotes the flow of Qi

Additionally in interval:
UB. 15 Xinshu – Shu point of the heart
UB. 17 Geshu – influential point for blood,
eliminates blood stagnation
He. 7 Shenmen – calms the heart
Sp. 6 Sanyinjiao – strengthens Yin and blood

References

1. Cheng Xinnong (1987) Chinese acupuncture an Moxibustion. Foreign Language Press, Beijing
2. Ellis A, Wisemann N, Boss K (1988) Fundamental of Chinese acupuncture. Paradigm Publications, Brookline/MA
3. Heinke W (1987) Kursskript und Kursnotizen, Kurse für Traditionelle Chinesische Medizin. Düsseldorf
4. Kapchuck T (1983) Chinese medicine. The web that has no weaver. Rider, London
5. Li Xiao Hai (1988) Kursskript und Kursnotizen, Traditionelle Syndrome. Düsseldorf
6. McDonald J (1987) Zang Fu Syndromes. NSW College of Natural Therapy, Sydney
7. O'Connor J, Bensky D (1981) Acupuncture – A Comprehensive Text. Eastland Press, Chicago
8. Ross J (1985) Zang Fu, the organ systems of traditional Chinese medicine. Churchill Livingstone, Edingburgh
9. Stux G (1994) Grundlagen der Akupunktur, 3rd edn. Springer, Berlin Heidelberg New York
10. Stux G, Stiller N, Pomeranz B (1994) Akupunktur – Lehrbuch und Atlas, 4th edn. Springer, Berlin Heidelberg New York
11. Wiseman N, Ellis A (1985) Fundamentals of Chinese medicine. Paradigm Publications, Brookline

9 Additional Methods of Treatment

In addition to acupuncture, moxibustion, laser acupuncture, and herbal treatment, new modalities and methods have been introduced to intensify the action of these traditional methods in chronic conditions. In this chapter new forms of treatment are presented, which focus more deeply and directly on the energy bases of therapy.

Chakra acupuncture, which is presented first, integrates the Indian chakra system, a system of major energy centers, into the acupuncture practice promoting and deepening the flow of Qi.

Awareness release technique (ART) is a new method to focus the conscious awareness into the blockages or stagnant areas and dissolve them. It is used in combination with acupuncture to release especially chronic stagnations, for example, in severe pain conditions and in diseases with diffuse symptoms.

Both methods are characterized by an intensive cooperation of the patient in the treatment process, thus taking more responsibility for the treatment results.

9.1 Chakra Acupuncture

Chakra acupuncture is an expansion of the practice of traditional Chinese acupuncture. Chakra acupuncture deepens the application of traditional acupuncture by including the Indian chakra system, a system of seven major energy centers.

The chakras of Indian medicine are energy centers. Seven main energy centers are known in the midline of the body, from the perineum to the cranium (Fig. 1). In addition, there are some dozens of minor energy centers of secondary importance, which in most cases correspond to the location of important acupuncture points. The chakras, similar to the Chinese organs, have certain functions.

The aim of the treatment in traditional Chinese acupuncture is to harmonize the flow of Qi by dissolving the blockages and stagnations in the channels and organs. Conditions of excess or deficiency are balanced, and thus achieving an undisturbed function of the organs by harmonizing Yin and Yang. These ideas are the basis of traditional Chinese acupuncture.

Chakra acupuncture extends and deepens the traditional application of acupuncture by including the Indian chakra system into the diagnosis and treatment. In chakra acupuncture, apart from the acupuncture points selected according to Chinese aspects, further *chakra points* are needled in the area of the seven energy centers. Thus the chakras are activated, and the energy flow is promoted; this is called *opening of the chakras.*

The most frequently used chakra points are Du 20 Baihui, which is situated in the center of the *crown chakra,* the 7th chakra, and Ex. 6 Sishencong surrounding Baihui. Other important chakra points are Ex. 1 Yintang and Du 15 Yamen for the sixth chakra, Ren 17 Shanzhong and Du 11 Shendao for the heart chakra.

After all acupuncture points have been needled with the usual technique, including traditionally chosen points and chakra points, the patient is asked *to direct his awareness* towards the relevant chakra (for example, towards the crown, where the points Du 20 Baihui and Ex. 6 Sishencong have been needled). Thus besides needling of the chakra points, *the focusing of the conscious awareness* i.e., the attention of the patient towards the respective chakra region, is important for the efficacy of the treatment.

After a short time the patient feels a sensation of a slight tingling or of a gentle flow in this area. The patient should observe this sensations during the whole course of the treatment session. The therapist, *together* with the patient, focuses his attention on this region too. He asks the patient repeatedly to be aware here, to "open this area" and to "let the energy flow from above downwards." If the opening of the chakra is not experienced by the patient in the beginning, the therapist asks the patient to breath into this area,

i. e., focusing his breath into the chakra. Thereby the opening of the chakra as well as the flow of life force in the crown energy center are intensified.

When the flow through one energy center is clearly experienced by the patient, one proceeds to the next energy center (for example, to the heart chakra in the center of the thorax). Here the points Ren 17 Shanzhong and Ren 15 Jiuwei have already been needled. The patient is then asked to breath into this area, to hold his awareness there, and to "open the heart chakra" until he feels a sensation of width, charge, and flow in this region.

The *first step* is to open the energy centers and to promote the flow of life force in them, establishing a strong charge, thus raising the awareness of the patient for the energy centers and vitalizing his energies. *At the beginning* of the chakra acupuncture treatment it is important to focus upon the *crown and the heart energy centers* and to establish a strong flow. The heart chakra, as the fourth, is situated in the center; above and below there are three chakras. Thus the heart chakra because of its midposition has an important harmonizing function for the whole energy of the body. Also, the healing quality of the heart harmonizes the other energy centers.

The *second step* is to focus the therapy on the blockages and stagnations causing the diseases and to dissolve them.

After a few treatment sessions, when the flow of energy in these chakras is well established, one proceeds to further chakras, especially to those where the illness of the patient is located. It is not recommended to start with the disturbed region, but to open and activate at first the main chakras (crown, heart, and base).

Description of the Chakras and their Relation to Acupuncture Points and Chinese Organs

1. Chakra   Base Chakra   Muladhara

Location: The first chakra is situated on the perineum and opens downwards. The position corresponds to the point Ren 1 Huiyin, the meeting point of the entire Yin.
Functions: The Yin corresponds to earth and thus the base chakra provides the energetic connection of the human being to the earth.

The opening of the base chakra and the energetic flow through the chakra is responsible for the energetic connection of the body to the earth, which is called grounding. This chakra corresponds to the kidney Yin.

Acupuncture point: Ren 1 Huiyin

2. Chakra   Polarity Chakra   Svadhishthana

Location: The second chakra is situated in the pelvis and has two openings, one forwards to the acupuncture points Ren 2–Ren 4 Guanyuan and one backwards to the sacrum, Du 2–Du 4 Mingmen.

Functions: The polarity chakra balances the Yin and Yang inside and outside; it forms the base for harmonious sexuality, i. e., the Yin and Yang balance outside. The first and second chakra correspond to the lower Jiao of the Sanjiao (pelvis). The polarity chakra corresponds to the kidney Yang, the urinary bladder and the large intestine.

Acupuncture points: Front: Ren 2 Qugu till Ren 4 Guanyuan
Back: Du 2 Yaoshu till Du 4 Mingmen

3. Chakra   Solar Plexus Chakra   Manipura

Location: The third chakra is situated in the abdomen. It opens forwards to the navel and backwards to the region of Du 5–Du 6.

Functions: The Manipura chakra regulates the personal will in the upper part and emotional expression in the lower part. In case of imbalance it is responsible for striving for power, anger, rage, and addiction.

The Chinese organs spleen and liver correspond to the third chakra. There is also a relation to the middle Jiao of the Sanjiao.

Acupuncture points: Ren 8 Shenjue, Ren 12 Zhongwan
Du 5 Xuanshu, Du 6 Jizhong

4. Chakra   Heart Chakra   Anahata

Location: The fourth chakra is situated in the center of the thorax and opens forwards to the point Ren 17 Shanzhong and backwards to the point Du 11 Shendao.

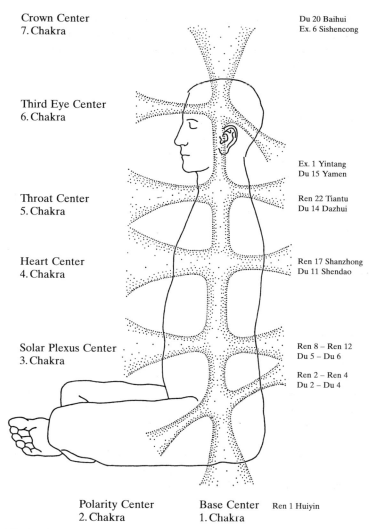

Crown Center
7. Chakra

Du 20 Baihui
Ex. 6 Sishencong

Third Eye Center
6. Chakra

Ex. 1 Yintang
Du 15 Yamen

Throat Center
5. Chakra

Ren 22 Tiantu
Du 14 Dazhui

Heart Center
4. Chakra

Ren 17 Shanzhong
Du 11 Shendao

Solar Plexus Center
3. Chakra

Ren 8 – Ren 12
Du 5 – Du 6

Ren 2 – Ren 4
Du 2 – Du 4

Polarity Center
2. Chakra

Base Center
1. Chakra

Ren 1 Huiyin

Fig. 1. Chakras and Chakrapoints

Functions: The corresponding functions are friendliness, understanding, compassion, balancing of contrasts, striving for harmony, inner peace, and love. The heart chakra, as the fourth chakra, represents the center of the human being, and it is the most important integrating chakra located between the three upper and the three lower chakras.

The Anahata chakra corresponds to the heart and the upper Jiao.

Acupuncture points: Ren 17 Shanzhong, Du 11 Shendao

5. Chakra   Throat Chakra   Vishuddha

Location: The fifth chakra is situated in the throat and opens forwards to the larynx and backwards to the point Du 14 Dazhui.

Functions: The throat chakra produces the strength and expressiveness of speech. Another function is creativity.

The throat chakra corresponds to the lung.

Acupuncture points: Ren 22 Tiantu, Du 14 Dazhui

6. Chakra   Third Eye   Ajna

Location: The sixth chakra is situated at the base of the skull. It opens forwards to the point Extra 1 Yintang and backwards to the point Du 15 Yamen.

Functions: The functions of the *Third Eye* are the ability to focus the mind, understanding, the power of discernment, intuition, and clairvoyance.

Acupuncture points: Ex.1 Yintang, Du 15 Yamen

7. Chakra   Crown Chakra   Sahasrara

Location: The seventh chakra is situated upon the cranium. It corresponds to the point Du 20 Baihui and Extra 6 Sishencong and opens upwards, like a crown.

Functions: The crown chakra represents the highest Yang in the body, in contrast to the meeting point of the entire Yin in the base

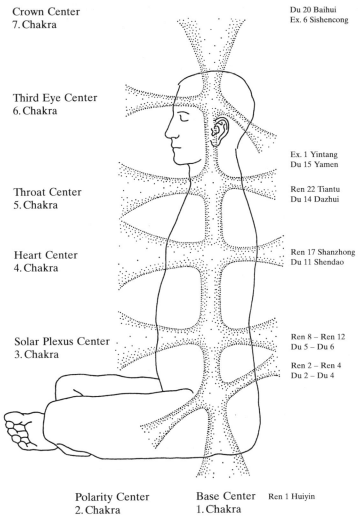

Crown Center
7. Chakra

Du 20 Baihui
Ex. 6 Sishencong

Third Eye Center
6. Chakra

Ex. 1 Yintang
Du 15 Yamen

Throat Center
5. Chakra

Ren 22 Tiantu
Du 14 Dazhui

Heart Center
4. Chakra

Ren 17 Shanzhong
Du 11 Shendao

Solar Plexus Center
3. Chakra

Ren 8 – Ren 12
Du 5 – Du 6

Ren 2 – Ren 4
Du 2 – Du 4

Polarity Center
2. Chakra

Base Center
1. Chakra

Ren 1 Huiyin

Fig. 1. Chakras and Chakrapoints

chakra. The crown chakra is considered to be responsible for the understanding of higher aspects of life, it provides the connection to the spiritual world. The point Du 20 Baihui as well as the Ex. 6 Sishencong are particularly important acupuncture points and serve to harmonize mental functions and the whole energy balance of the body.

Acupuncture points: Du 20 Baihui, Ex. 6 Sishencong

9.2 Awareness Release Technique, ART

An important method to clear blockages and stagnated areas is ART developed by Robert T. Jaffe. It is often used together with acupuncture in severe and chronic diseases to enhance the action of conventional acupuncture and to bring more conscious awareness into the diseased region.

In contrast to Western medicine, where pain and other uncomfortable symptoms are repressed by analgesic or spasmolytic drugs, direct methods of "energy medicine" focus the attention of the patient onto the diseased area and thus bring the consciousness in it.

Before starting with ART the patient is needled as usual and with closed eyes relaxes and directs his focus into his body.

Awareness release technique has four steps:

1. **Awareness.** The patient focuses on his problem, pain, region of nervousness, or anxiety (i.e., the blockage of energy). He communicates his present problem to the therapist.
2. **Identification.** The second step is a more precise and detailed identification of the problem. The therapist asks the patient to focus more deeply on the region of the blockage to visualize it, *describing its location, size, borders, density, temperature and colour.* Later the awareness is also directed to the emotions related to the blockage and the thoughts arising from it. During the second step of ART through precise visualisation, the awareness goes deeper into the blockage.

3. **Release or transformation** of the blocked or stagnated energy. During this step the patient's conscious awareness transforms the density of the blockage or releases its charge completely.

   This is done by a deepening of the focus through *breathing consciously* into the blockage by the patient. The therapist also directes his attention onto the problem of the patient and observes changes in the energy pattern of the blockage. If the patient becomes tired or does not breath intensively into the area of the blockage, the therapist asks the patient to deepen the breath. Persistent deepening and focusing of the breath into the blockage releases it generally during the acupuncture session within 10–20 min.

4. **Integration.** In the fourth step the flow of life force through the affected area is reestablished and harmonized. This is generally achieved during the treatment session, but perhaps later at home by the patient himself by bringing his awareness repeatedly into the affected area and promoting the flow.

   ART is an excellent method to dissolve blockages which are very severe, especially those in which acupuncture treatment alone does not achieve satisfactory results.

Bibliography

1. Jaffe RT (1990) Energy mastery seminars, course script, Sedona
2. Jung CG (1948) Über psychische Energie und das Wesen der Träume. Rascher, Zürich
3. Krieger D (1979) The therapeutic touch, how to use hands to help to heal. Pentrice Hall, New York
4. Stux G (1994) Einführung in die Akupunktur. 4th edn. Springer, Berlin Heidelberg New York
5. Stux G (1992) Akupunktur und A.R.T. Therapeutikon 6/1–2: 42–43
6. Stux G (1992) Was ist Energie-Medizin? Therapeutikon 6/4: 171–172
7. Stux G (1994) Was ist Energie-Medizin? Therapiewoche 44/28: 1620–1624
8. Stux G (1995) Chakra Flow Meditation. Therapeutikon (in preparation)

Appendix A
World Health Organization
List of Indications for Acupuncture

G. STUX

Respiratory tract disorders

Acute sinusitis
Acute rhinitis
Common cold
Acute tonsillitis

Bronchopulmonary disorders

Acute bronchitis
Bronchial asthma
(most effective in children and in patients
without concomitant diseases)

Disorders of the eye

Acute conjunctivitis
Central retinitis
Myopia (in children)
Cataract (without complications)

Disorders of the mouth cavity

Toothache
Pain after tooth extraction
Gingivitis
Acute and chronic pharyngitis

Gastrointestinal disorders

Spasm of the oesophagus and cardia

Hiccoughs
Gastroptosis
Acute and chronic gastritis
Gastric hyperacidity
Chronic duodenal ulcer
Acute and chronic colitis
Acute bacterial dysentery
Constipation
Diarrhea
Paralytic ileus

Neurological and orthopedic disorders

Headache
Migraine
Trigeminal neuralgia
Facial paralysis
Paralysis after apoplectic fit
Peripheral neuropathy
Paralysis caused by poliomyelitis
Ménière's syndrome
Neurogenic bladder dysfunction
Nocturnal enuresis
Intercostal neuralgia
Periarthritis humeroscapularis
Tennis elbow
Sciatica, lumbar pain
Rheumatoid arthritis

Appendix B
Nomenclature and Abbreviations for Channels and Points

Main channels (Jing)	Abbreviations used	
	In this volume	**Elsewhere in the literature**
Lung channel, Shou Tai Yin	**Lu.**	LU, P
Large intestine channel, Shou Yang Ming	**LI.**	L.I., Co, IG
Stomach channel, Zu Yang Ming	**St.**	S, ST, V
Spleen channel, Zu Tai Yin	**Sp.**	LP
Heart channel, Shou Shao Yin	**He.**	H., Ht, C
Small intestine channel, Shou Tai Yang	**SI.**	S.I., IT
Urinary bladder channel, Zu Tai Yang	**UB.**	U.B., B, Bl, VU
Kidney channel, Zu Shao Yin	**Ki.**	K., KID, R
Pericardium channel, Shou Jue Yin	**Pe.**	P., HC, TW
Sanjiao channel, Shou Shao Yang	**SJ.**	S.J., TB, TH, SC
Gallbladder channel, Zu Shao Yang	**GB.**	G.B., VF
Liver channel, Zu Jue Yin	**Liv.**	Li, LIV, H

8 Extraordinary channels,
"irregular or marvellous channels," Qi Jingba Mai

Du Mai, governing vessel	**Du**	Gv, GV, TM
Ren Mai, conceptional vessel	**Ren**	Co, CV, JM

Chong Mai (Chung Mo) Penetrating vessel
Dai Mai (Tai Mo) Belt or Girdle vessel
Yangqiao, Yang Chiao, (Yang Keo), Yang motility or ankle vessel
Yinqiao, Yin Chiao, (Yin Keo), Yin motility or ankle vessel
Yangwei, Yang regulating, linking or reuniting channel
Yinwei, Yin regulating, linking or reuniting channel

12 Jingbie, distinct or divergent channels
(separate master meridian)
12 Jingjing, tendinomuscular channels

Points

Shu point, Beishu, or back transport point, Back Shu point (Yu)
Mu or alarm point, front collecting point (Mo)
Influential point, gathering point, Hui Xue
Xi-cleft point, accumulation point (Tsri)
Five Shu points, five transporting points Wushu, Shu I-V (Yu)
Tonification point
Sedative point
Jing well point, Shu I (Ting)
Ying point, Ying spring point, Shu II (Yong, Rong)
Shu stream point, Shu III (Yu)
Yuan source point (Yunn)
Jing point, Jing river point, Shu IV (King)
He point, He Sea point, Shu V (He)
Luo connecting point (Lo)
Confluent point, key point

Wade-Giles transcription is given in parentheses.

Appendix C
Glossary of Chinese Terms

陽	**Yang**	consists of the two ideograms:
阜=阝	**fu**	for hill and
昜	**yang**	for brightness, expansiveness

Yang is the light side of the hill, the sunny side.

陰	**Yin**	consists of two ideograms:
今	**jin**	now or present and
云	**yun**	for clouds

Yin is the shady side (cloudy side) of the hill. Yin and Yang are the complementary polar forces, which are continuously transformed.

According to Chinese philosophy the transformation is accomplished in **five phases, wu xing.**

五 行

五	**Wu**	is the ideogram for 5
行	**Xing**	means to go, the journey, the change, to take place, and consists of two ideograms:
彳	**chi**	means small step and
亍	**chu**	to go to

According to Chinese philosophy the five phases make up a complex system which explains the phases of phenomena and the correlations with the physical world. In medicine the five phases classify the physiological and pathological relations of the internal organs, tissues, and sense organs.

氣	**Qi**	consists of two ideograms:
气	**qi**	for air, vapor, or breathing, and the ideogram
米	**mi**	for rice or grain

Qi is the vital energy and is symbolized by two parts of the ideogram: air, for breathing, and grain as the origin of nutrition. These form the basis of vital energy: breathing and nutrition.
mi, the grain, also symbolizes the vital energy latent in a grain of seed.
In the ancient literature qi is also written as fire – **luo** – instead of grain.

示申	**Shen**	consists of two ideograms:
示	**shi**	to make known, to point at, to show and
申	**shen**	to report

Shen means spirit, psychic energy, reasoning ability, consciousness. The original meaning of shen, certainly stemming from the time of ancestor worship, was the communication between man and gods by way of the spirits.

| 米青 | **Jing** | consists of two ideograms: |
| 米 | **mi** | for grain and |

青	qing	for fresh or young
	Jing	is the life essence, the subtle material, the material basis of Qi, the vital energy. The "young" grain here symbolizes the essence of life.
血	Xue	means blood. It is composed of two ideograms:
	chu	for drop or point and
血	min	for vessel
臟,腑	Zang and fu	designate the Chinese internal organs.
腑	Fu	are the Yang organs, such as stomach, large intestine, and gallbladder. The ideogram consists of two parts:
肉=月	rou	for flesh and
府	fu	for prefecture, official residence

The ideogram for rou is found in the character used for all internal organs. Fu organs, as governing authorities, influence the connected Yin organs.

臟	Zang	consists of the two ideograms:
月	rou	flesh and
藏	zang	to hide, to preserve, to store

The Zang organs are the Yin organs, such as lung, liver, and spleen. According to traditional Chinese thinking the Zang organs store the vital energy. These organs are hidden deep within the body.

經 絡   **Jing luo**   is the Chinese designation for the system of channels and collaterals (Jing are the channels, Luo are the collaterals).

經   The original meaning of the ideogram **jing** is the warp threads in weaving. The longitudinal threads provide the structure of the woven fabric as the channels are the structural elements of the body.

絡   **Luo**   means to connect, to knot. The Luo vessels connect the coupled channels (Jing) with each other.

Appendix D
Alphabetic List of Chinese Point Names

Anmian I	Ex.	8	Chongyang	St.	42	Erbai	Ex.	24
Anmian II	Ex.	9	Ciliao	UB.	32	Erjian	LI.	2
						Ermen	SJ.	21
Bafeng	Ex.	36	Dabao	Sp.	21			
Baihuanshu	UB.	30	Dachangshu	UB.	25	Feishu	UB.	13
Baihui	Du	20	Dadu	Sp.	2	Feiyang	UB.	58
Baohuang	UB.	53	Dadun	Liv.	1	Fengchi	GB.	20
Baxie	Ex.	28	Dahe	Ki.	12	Fengfu	Du	16
Benshen	GB.	13	Daheng	Sp.	15	Fenglong	St.	40
Biguan	St.	31	Daimai	GB.	26	Fengmen	UB.	12
Binao	LI.	14	Daju	St.	27	Fengshi	GB.	31
Bingfeng	SI.	12	Daling	Pe.	7	Fuai	Sp.	16
Bizhong	Ex.	23	Dannang	Ex.	35	Fubai	GB.	10
Bulang	Ki.	22	Danshu	UB.	19	Fufen	UB.	41
Burong	St.	19	Dashu	UB.	11	Fujie	Sp.	14
			Daying	St.	5	Fuliu	Ki.	7
Changqiang	Du	1	Dazhong	Ki.	4	Fushe	Sp.	13
Chengfu	UB.	36	Dazhui	Du	14	Futu (femur)	St.	32
Cheng-	UB.	6	Dicang	St.	4	Futu (neck)	LI.	18
guang			Diji	Sp.	8	Fuxi	UB.	38
Chengjiang	Ren	24	Dingchuan	Ex.	17	Fuyang	UB.	59
Chengjin	UB.	56	Diwuhui	GB.	42			
Chengling	GB.	18	Dubi	St.	35	Ganshu	UB.	18
Chengman	St.	20	Duiduan	Du	27	Gaohuang	UB.	43
Chengqi	St.	1	Dushu	UB.	16	Geguan	UB.	46
Chengshan	UB.	57				Geshu	UB.	17
Chize	Lu.	5				Gongsun	Sp.	4
Chongmen	Sp.	12				Guanchong	SJ.	1

Guangming	GB. 37	Jianzhong	Ex. 22	Ligou	Liv. 5
Guanmen	St. 22	Jianzhong-shu	SI. 15	Lingdao	He. 4
Guanyuan	Ren 4			Linghou	Ex. 34
Guanyuan-shu	UB. 26	Jiaosun	SJ. 20	Lingtai	Du 10
		Jiaoxin	Ki. 8	Lingxu	Ki. 24
Guilai	St. 29	Jiexi	St. 41	Linqi (foot)	GB. 41
		Jimai	Liv. 12	Linqi (head)	GB. 15
Hanyan	GB. 4	Jimen	Sp. 11	Lougu	Sp. 7
Heding	Ex. 31	Jingbi	Ex. 13	Luoque	UB. 8
Hegu	LI. 4	Jinggu	UB. 64	Luozhen	Ex. 26
Heliao (ear)	SJ. 22	Jingmen	GB. 25	Luxi	SJ. 19
Heliao (nose)	LI. 19	Jingming	UB. 1		
		Jingqu	Lu. 8	Meichong	UB. 3
Henggu	Ki. 11	Jinjin, Yuye	Ex. 10	Mingmen	Du 4
Heyang	UB. 55	Jinmen	UB. 63	Muchuang	GB. 16
Houding	Du 19	Jinsuo	Du 8		
Houxi	SI. 3	Jiquan	He. 1	Naohu	Du 17
Huagai	Ren 20	Jiuwei	Ren 15	Naohui	SJ. 13
Huangmen	UB. 51	Jizhong	Du 6	Naokong	GB. 19
Huangshu	Ki. 16	Jueyinshu	UB. 14	Naoshu	SI. 10
Huantiao	GB. 30	Juliao (femur)	GB. 29	Neiguan	Pe. 6
Huaroumen	St. 24			Neiting	St. 44
Huatuojiaji	Ex. 21	Juliao (nose)	St. 3		
Huiyang	UB. 35			Pangguang-shu	UB. 28
Huiyin	Ren 1	Jugu	LI. 16		
Huizong	SJ. 7	Juque	Ren 14	Pianli	LI. 6
Hunmen	UB. 47			Pishu	UB. 20
		Kongzui	Lu. 6	Pohu	UB. 42
Jiache	St. 6	Kufang	St. 14	Pushen	UB. 61
Jiacheng-jiang	Ex. 5	Kunlun	UB. 60		
				Qianding	Du 21
Jianjing	GB. 21	Lanwei	Ex. 33	Qiangjian	Du 18
Jianli	Ren 11	Laogong	Pe. 8	Qiangu	SI. 2
Jianliao	SJ. 14	Liangmen	St. 21	Qiaoyin (foot)	GB. 44
Jianshi	Pe. 5	Liangqiu	St. 34		
Jianwaishu	SI. 14	Lianquan	Ren 23	Qiaoyin (head)	GB. 11
Jianyu	LI. 15	Lidui	St. 45		
Jianzhen	SI. 9	Lieque	Lu. 7	Qichong	St. 30

Qihai	Ren	6	Shangliao	UB.	31	Siman	Ki. 14
Qihaishu	UB.	24	Shangqiu	Sp.	5	Sishencong	Ex. 6
Qihu	St.	13	Shangqu	Ki.	17	Sizhukong	SJ. 23
Qimai	SJ.	18	Shangwan	Ren	13	Suliao	Du 25
Qimen	Liv.	14	Shangxing	Du	23		
Qingleng-	SJ.	11	Shangyang	LI.	1	Taibai	Sp. 3
yuan			Shanzhong	Ren	17	Taichong	Liv. 3
Qingling	He.	2	Shaochong	He.	9	Taixi	Ki. 3
Qishe	St.	11	Shaofu	He.	8	Taiyang	Ex. 2
Qiuhou	Ex.	4	Shaohai	He.	3	Taiyi	St. 23
Qiuxu	GB.	40	Shaoshang	Lu.	11	Taiyuan	Lu. 9
Qixue	Ki.	13	Shaoze	SI.	1	Taodao	Du 13
Quanliao	SI.	18	Shencang	Ki.	25	Tianchi	Pe. 1
Qubin	GB.	7	Shendao	Du	11	Tianchong	GB. 9
Quchai	UB.	4	Shenfeng	Ki.	23	Tianchuang	SI. 16
Quchi	LI.	11	Shenmai	UB.	62	Tianding	LI. 17
Quepen	St.	12	Shenmen	He.	7	Tianfu	Lu. 3
Qugu	Ren	2	Shenque	Ren	8	Tianjing	SJ. 10
Ququan	Liv.	8	Shenshu	UB.	23	Tianliao	SJ. 15
Quyuan	SI.	13	Shentang	UB.	44	Tianquan	Pe. 2
Quze	Pe.	3	Shenting	Du	24	Tianrong	SI. 17
			Shenzhu	Du	12	Tianshu	St. 25
Rangu	Ki.	2	Shidou	Sp.	17	Tiantu	Ren 22
Renying	St.	9	Shiguan	Ki.	18	Tianxi	Sp. 18
Renzhong	Du	26	Shimen	Ren	5	Tianyou	SJ. 16
Riyue	GB.	24	Shiqizhui	Ex.	19	Tianzhu	UB. 10
Rugen	St.	18	Shixuan	Ex.	30	Tianzong	SI. 11
Ruzhong	St.	17	Shousanli	LI.	10	Tiaokou	St. 38
			Shuaigu	GB.	8	Tinggong	SI. 19
Sanjian	LI.	3	Shufu	Ki.	27	Tinghui	GB. 2
Sanjiaoshu	UB.	22	Shugu	UB.	65	Tonggu	UB. 66
Sanyangluo	SJ.	8	Shuidao	St.	28	(foot)	
Sanyinjiao	Sp.	6	Shuifen	Ren	9	Tonggu	Ki. 20
Shangguan	GB.	3	Shuiquan	Ki.	5	(thorax)	
Shangjuxu	St.	37	Shuitu	St.	10	Tongli	He. 5
Shanglian	LI.	9	Sibai	St.	2	Tongtian	UB. 7
Shanglian-	Ex.	12	Sidu	SJ.	9	Tongziliao	GB. 1
quan			Sifeng	Ex.	29	Touwei	St. 8

Waiguan	SJ.	5
Wailing	St.	26
Waiqiu	GB.	36
Wangu (hand)	SI.	4
Wangu (head)	GB.	12
Weibao	Ex.	15
Weicang	UB.	50
Weidao	GB.	28
Weishang	Ex.	14
Weishu	UB.	21
Weiyang	UB.	39
Weizhong	UB.	40
Wenliu	LI.	7
Wuchu	UB.	5
Wuli (hand)	LI.	13
Wuli (femur)	Liv.	10
Wuming	Ex.	18
Wushu	GB.	27
Wuyi	St.	15
Xiabai	Lu.	4
Xiaguan	St.	7
Xiajuxu	St.	39
Xialian	LI.	8
Xialiao	UB.	34
Xiangu	St.	43
Xiaochang-shu	UB.	27
Xiaohai	SI.	8
Xiaoluo	SJ.	12
Xiawan	Ren	10
Xiaxi	GB.	43
Xiguan	Liv.	7
Ximen	Pe.	4
Xingjian	Liv.	2
Xinhui	Du	22
Xinshu	UB.	15
Xiongxiang	Sp.	19
Xiyan	Ex.	32
Xiyang-guan	GB.	33
Xuanji	Ren	21
Xuanli	GB.	6
Xuanlu	GB.	5
Xuanshu	Du	5
Xuanzhong	GB.	39
Xuehai	Sp.	10
Yamen	Du	15
Yangbai	GB.	14
Yangchi	SJ.	4
Yangfu	GB.	38
Yanggang	UB.	48
Yanggu	SI.	5
Yangjiao	GB.	35
Yanglao	SI.	6
Yangling-quan	GB.	34
Yangxi	LI.	5
Yaoqi	Ex.	20
Yaoshu	Du	2
Yaoyang-guan	Du	3
Yatong	Ex.	27
Yemen	SJ.	2
Yiteng	SJ.	17
Yiming	Ex.	7
Yinbai	Sp.	1
Yinbao	Liv.	9
Yindu	Ki.	19
Yingchuang	St.	16
Yingu	Ki.	10
Yingxiang	LI.	20
Yinjiao (abdomen)	Ren	7
Yinjiao (mouth)	Du	28
Yinlian	Liv.	11
Yinling-quan	Sp.	9
Yinmen	UB.	37
Yinshi	St.	33
Yintang	Ex.	1
Yinxi	He.	6
Yishe	UB.	49
Yixi	UB.	45
Yongquan	Ki.	1
Youmen	Ki.	21
Yuanye	GB.	22
Yuji	Lu.	10
Yunmen	Lu.	2
Yutang	Ren	18
Yuyao	Ex.	3
Yuzhen	UB.	9
Yuzhong	Ki.	26
Zanzhu	UB.	2
Zengyin	Ex.	11
Zhangmen	Liv.	13
Zhaohai	Ki.	6
Zhejin	GB.	23
Zhengying	GB.	17
Zhibian	UB.	54
Zhigou	SJ.	6
Zhishi	UB.	52
Zhiyang	Du	9
Zhiyin	UB.	67
Zhizheng	SI.	7
Zhongchong	Pe.	9
Zhongdu (femur)	GB.	32

Zhongdu (foot)	Liv.	6	Zhongshu	Du	7	Zhourong	Sp.	20
			Zhongting	Ren	16	Zhubin	Ki.	9
Zhongfeng	Liv.	4	Zhongwan	Ren	12	Zigong (abdomen)	Ex.	16
Zhongfu	Lu.	1	Zhongzhu (abdomen)	Ki.	15			
Zhongji	Ren	3				Zigong (thorax)	Ren	19
Zhongliao	UB.	33	Zhongzhu (hand)	SJ.	3	Zusanli	St.	36
Zhonglushu	UB.	29						
Zhongquan	Ex.	25	Zhouliao	LI.	12			

Bibliography

Academy of Traditional Chinese Medicine (1975) An outline of Chinese acupuncture. Foreign Language Press, Peking

Agrawal AL, Sharma GN (1980) Clinical practice of acupuncture. Acupuncture Foundation of India, Raipur

Anonymous (1980) Essentials of Chinese acupuncture. Foreign Languages Press, Beijing

Auerswald W, König GK (1982) Die neurochemische Basis der Akupunkturanalgesie. Maudrich, Vienna

Bachmann G (1959) Die Akupunktur – eine Ordnungstherapie. Haug, Heidelberg

Bannermann RH (1979) Akupunktur: Die Ansicht der WHO. Weltgesundheit-Magazin der WHO, 12

Becker-Carus C, Heyden T, Kelle A (1985) Die Wirksamkeit von Akupunktur und Einstellungs-Entspannungstraining zur Behandlung primärer Schlafstörungen. Klin Psych Psychopath Psychother 33/2: 161–172

Bischko J (1978) Akupunktur für Fortgeschrittene. Haug, Heidelberg

Bischko J (1979) Einführung in die Akupunktur. Haug, Heidelberg

Bonica JJ (1974) Therapeutical acupuncture in the P. R. China, implications for American medicine. JAMA 228: 1544–1551

Bunzel B, Riegler R, Pfersmann C (1986) Schmerz bei chronischer Mastopathie. Verbesserung der subjektiven Empfindungen nach Akupunktur. Klinikarzt 15/6: 428–440

China Association of Acupuncture and Moxibustion (1986) Brief explanation of point names of 14 meridians. Journal of Traditional Chinese Medicine 6/1: 57–68, 6/2

Cignolini A (1986) Discussion on semantics. Journal of Traditional Chinese Medicine 6/3: 222–226

Dinstl K, Fischer PL (1981) Der Laser. Grundlagen der klinischen Anwendung. Springer, Berlin Heidelberg New York

Fernando F, Fernando L (1979) Theory and practice of traditional Chinese acupuncture. Acupuncture Foundation of Sri Lanka, Colombo

First World Conference on Acupuncture-Moxibustion (1987) World Federation of Acupuncture and Moxibustion Societies, Beijing

Fisch G (1979) Akupunktur. Goldmann, Munich

Fischl F (1984) Geburtshilfe und Frauenheilkunde 44: 510–512

Han JS (ed) (1987) The neurochemical basis of pain relief by acupuncture. A collection of papers 1973–1987 Beijing Medical University. China Publishing House, Beijing

Hastings AC, Fadiman J, Gordon JS (1980) Health for the whole person. Westview, Boulder

Herget HF, L Allemand H, Kalweit K (1976) Klinische Erfahrungen und erste Ergebnisse mit kombinierter Akupunktur-Analgesie bei offenen Herzoperationen am Zentrum für Chirurgie der Justus-Liebig-Universität Gießen. Anaesthesist 25: 223–230

Hu Bing (1982) A brief introduction of the science of breathing exercise. Hai Teng, Hong Kong

Jayasuriya A (1979) Clinical acupuncture. Acupuncture Foundation of Sri Lanka, Colombo

Jayasuriya A (1981) Textbook of acupuncture science. Acupuncture Foundation of Sri Lanka, Colombo

Jayasuriya A, Fernando F (1978) Theory and practise of scientific acupuncture. Lake House, Colombo

Jayaweera B (1981) Auriculotherapy. Acupuncture Foundation of Sri Lanka, Colombo

Jia LH, Jia ZX (1986) Pointing therapy – a Chinese traditional therapeutic skill. Shandong Science and Technology Press, Jinan

Kaptchuk TJ (1983) Chinese Medicine, the web that has no weaver. Hutchinson, London

Kleinkort JA, Foley RA (1984) Laser acupuncture, its use in physical therapy. Am J Acupuncture 12/1: 5156

König G, Wancura I (1978) Einführung in die chinesische Ohrakupunktur. Haug, Heidelberg

König G, Wancura I (1979) Praxis und Theorie der neuen chinesischen Akupunktur, vol I. Maudrich, Vienna

König G, Wancura I (1984) Praxis und Theorie der neuen chinesischen Akupunktur, vol II. Maudrich, Vienna

Kovinskii IT (1973) The treatment of burns by laser. Zdravoorkhr Kaz 3: 46

Kwong LC (1976) Nose, hand and foot acupuncture. Commercial Press, Hong Kong

Maciocia G (1989) The foundations of Chinese medicine, a comprehensive text for acupuncturists and herbalists. Churchill Livingstone, Edinburgh

Mann F (1976) The meridians of acupuncture. Heinemann, London

Mann F (1978) Acupuncture. Heinemann, London

Marx HG (1979) Anwendung der Akupunktur in einer Fachklinik für Suchtkranke. Wien Z Suchtforsch 2/3: 45–46

McDonald J (1985) Zang fu syndromes. Sidney

McDonald J (1986) Acupuncture point dynamics. Sidney

Mester E (1975) Clinical results of wound-healing stimulation with laser and experimental studies of the action mechanism. Laser' 75 Opto-Electronics Conference Proceedings. IPC Science and Technology Press, Guildford

Mester E (1977) Neuere Untersuchungen über die Wirkung der Laser-strahlen auf die Wundheilung. Laser' 77 Opto-Electronics Conference Proceedings. Ipc Science and Technology Press, Guildford

Mester E, Ludany G, Sellyei M, Szende B, Gyenes G (1968) Untersuchungen über die hemmende, bzw. fördernde Wirkung der Laserstrahlen. Arch Klin Chir 322: 1022

Mester E, Ludany G, Frenyo V, Sellyei M, Szende B (1971) Experimental and clinical observations with laser. Panminerva Med 13: 538

Mester E, Szende B, Spiry T, Scher A (1972) Stimulation of wound healing by laser rays. Acta Chir Acad Sci Hung 13: 315

Mester E, Bacsy E, Korenyi-Both A, Kovacs I, Spiry T (1974) Klinische, elektronenoptische und enzymhistochemische Untersuchungen über die Wirkung der Laserstrahlen auf die Wundheilung. Langenbecks Arch Chir [Suppl Chir Forum] 1974: 261

Mester E, Jaszsagi-Nagy E, Hamar M (1974) Der Einfluß von Laserstrah-lung auf stimulierte menschliche Lymphozyten. Radiobiol Radiother 15–767

Mester E, Korenyi-Both A, Spiry T, Scher A, Tisza S (1974) Neuere Unter-suchungen über die Laserstrahlen auf die Wundheilung. Z Exp Chir [Suppl] 7: 9–17

Mester E, Nagylucskay S, Mester A (1977) Wirkungen der direkten Laser-bestrahlung auf menschliche immunkomponente Zellen. Laser + Elek-tro-Optik 1: 40

Mehta M (1978) Alternative methods of treating pain. Anaesthesia 33/3: 258–263

Melzack R, Wall PD (1965) Pain mechanism: a new theory. Science 150: 971–979

Molsberger A (1988) Die Therapie der akuten und chronischen Epicondy-litis humeri lateralis (Tennisarm) mit Akupunktur. In: Spintge R, Droh R (eds) Schmerz und Sport. Springer, Berlin Heidelberg New York

National Symposium of Acupuncture, Moxibustion and Acupuncture An-aesthesia (1979) Collection of 534 abstracts of latest research papers. Foreign Language Press, Beijing

Needham J (1956) Science and Civilization in China. History of Scientific Thought. Cambridge University Press, Cambridge

Needham J, Gwei-Djen L (1980) Celestial lancets – a history and rationale of acupuncture and moxibustion. Cambridge University Press, Cambridge

O Connor J, Bensky D (1981) Acupuncture. A comprehensive text. Shang-hai College of Traditional Medicine. Eastland, Chicago

Palos S (1984) Consilium cedip. acupunturae. Therapie in Wort und Bild. CEDIP, Munich

Pongratz W, Linke W, Baum M, Richter JA (1977) Elektroakupunktur-An-algesie bei 500 herzchirurgischen Eingriffen. Tierärztl Prax 5/4: 545–558

Popp FA, Becker G, König HL, Peschka W (1979) Electromagnetic bio-in-formation. Proceedings of the symposium. Urban and Schwarzenberg, Munich

Porkert E (1976) Lehrbuch der chinesischen Diagnostik. Fischer, Heidelberg

Pothmann R, Yeh HL (1982) The effects of treatment with antibiotics, laser and acupuncture upon chronic maxillary sinusitis in children. Am Chin Med 10: 55–58

Pothmann R, Stux G, Weigel A (1980) Frozen shoulder: differential acupuncture therapy with point St.38. Am J Acupunct 8/1: 65–69

Richardson PH, Vincent CA (1986) Acupuncture for the treatment of pain: a review of evaluative research. Pain 24: 15–40

Ross J (1985) Zang fu. Churchill Livingstone, Edinburgh

Schmidt H (1979) Akupunkturtherapie nach der chinesischen Typenlehre. Hippokrates, Stuttgart

Schnorrenberger CC (1979) Lehrbuch der chinesischen Medizin für westliche Ärzte. Hippokrates, Stuttgart

Second National Symposium of Acupuncture and Moxibustion and Acupuncture Anaestesia (1984) All-China Society of Acupuncture and Moxibustion, Beijing

Stiefvater EW (1978) Praxis der Akupunktur. Fischer, Heidelberg

Stux G (1982) Basic acupuncture video teaching films in 8 lectures. Paramed, Augsburg

Stux G (1984) Acupressure and moxibustion. Video teaching film in 2 lectures. Düsseldorf

Stux G (1984) Treatment of migraine with acupuncture and moxibustion, pilot study on 50 patients. Second national symposium, Beijing

Stux G (1985) Akupressur und Moxibustion. Bergmann, Munich

Stux G (1994) Einführung in die Akupunktur. Springer, Berlin Heidelberg New York

Stux G, Stiller N, Pothmann R, Jayasuriya A (1981) Lehrbuch der klinischen Akupunktur. Springer, Berlin Heidelberg New York

Stux G, Jayasuriya A (1982) Atlas der Akupunktur. Springer, Berlin Heidelberg New York

Stux G, Mannheimer JS (1982) Therapie-Atlas Tenzcare. Optimale Stimulationsstellen für TENS-Elektroden. 3M Deutschland GmbH, Neuss

Stux G, Sahm KA (1986) Chinese Ideograms. A survey of terms in TCM. Br J Acupunct 9/2: 4–6

Stux G, Pomeranz B (1987) Acupuncture – textbook and atlas. Springer, Berlin Heidelberg New York

Stux G, Fernando F, Jayasuriya A (1979) Efficacy of acupuncture in spastic disorders of skeletal muscle. Am J Acupunct 7/2: 167–169

Stux G, Stiller N, Pomeranz B (1993) Akupunktur – Lehrbuch und Atlas. 4rd edn. Springer, Berlin Heidelberg New York

Tenk H (1978) Problematik der Akupunktur in der Kinderheilkunde. Haug, Heidelberg

Tiquia R (1986) Chinese infant massage. Greenhouse, Richmond

Unschuld PU (1980) Medizin in China. Eine Ideengeschichte. Beck, Munich

Unschuld PU (1986) Medicine in China. A history of pharmaceutics. University of California Press, Berkeley

Unschuld PU (1986) Nan-Ching. The classic of difficult issues. University of California Press, Berkeley

Van Nghi N (1975) Pathogenese und Pathologie der Energetik in der chinesischen Medizin. M.L. Verlag, Uelzen

Vincent CA, Richardson PH (1986) The evaluation of therapeutic acupuncture: concepts and methods. Pain 24: 1–13

Vinnemeier M (1978) Arbeitsmaterial zur Akupunktur. Eigenverlag, Velbert

Wall PD (1978) The gate control theory of pain mechanism, a reexamination and restatement. Brain 101: 1–18

Wang Xue Tai (1987) An illustrated history of acupuncture and moxibustion. Foreign Language Press, Beijing

Wiseman N, Ellis A (1985) Fundamentals of Chinese medicine. Paradigm, Brookline

Wu CC (1976) Preliminary report on effects of acupuncture on hyperlipidemia in man. Artery 2/2: 181–195

Wu CC, Hsu CJ (1979) Neurogenetic regulation of lipid metabolism in rabbits: a mechanism for cholesterol-lowering effect of acupuncture. Atherosclerosis 33/2: 153–164

Yau PS (1975) Scalp-needling therapy. Medicine and Health, Hong Kong

Zhang Xiangtong, HT Chang (1986) Research on acupuncture, moxibustion, and acupuncture anesthesia. Science Press, Beijing; Springer, Berlin Heidelberg New York

Zhang Zhongjing (1986) Treatise on febrile diseases caused by cold. New World Press, Beijing

Zhang Zhongjing (1987) Synopsis of prescriptions of the golden chamber. New World Press, Beijing

G. Stux, B. Pomeranz

Acupuncture
Textbook and Atlas

1987. UP **DM 154,-**; UP öS 1201,20; UP sFr 145,-
ISBN 3-540-17331-5

Following an introduction to the philosophical and
theoretical background of traditional Chinese medicine,
the diagnostic system is presented: the Chinese system of
channels and functional organs, the significance of points
and point categories, methods of needling and moxibustion. There is also a chapter on treatment based on
western diagnosis.

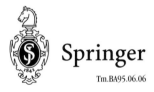

G. Stux

Acupuncture

Posters and Selector

1995. approx. **DM 24,80**; approx. öS 193,50;
approx. sFr 27,50 ISBN 3-540-59455-8

The posters and selector, part of *Stux, Acupuncture - Textbook and Atlas*, are now available separately. The most important acupuncture points are clearly depicted topographically on posters. We chose not to use photographs of the body surface because the structures which are directly under the skin cannot be portrayed. To ensure a clear and yet exact representation the bones have been drawn in the background. The graphic representation of the meridians and points are an indispensable aid to every acupuncturist, and the various categories of acupuncture points are presented in tables on the selector, enabling the user to recognize the most important points of a meridian at a glance.

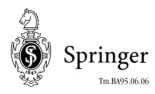

Tm.BA95.06.06

Springer-Verlag
and the Environment

We at Springer-Verlag firmly believe that an international science publisher has a special obligation to the environment, and our corporate policies consistently reflect this conviction.

We also expect our business partners – paper mills, printers, packaging manufacturers, etc. – to commit themselves to using environmentally friendly materials and production processes.

The paper in this book is made from low- or no-chlorine pulp and is acid free, in conformance with international standards for paper permanency.